CHOICES

Prevent Heart Attacks That
Begin in Childhood

CHOICES

Prevent Heart Attacks
That Begin in Childhood

Your Life & Health Depend on

Overcoming Stress,

Renewing Health and Relationships

Jack Dawson, MD

NightLight Publishing, Inc.

Atlanta, Georgia

NightLight Publishing, Inc.
P.O. Box 78504
Atlanta, Georgia 30357
www.nightlightpublishinginc.com

This book, CHOICES: Prevent Heart Attacks That Begin in Childhood, *is a platform for transformation and a guide for living.*

It is dedicated not only to children but also to the reader pursuing meaningful change.

CONTENTS

PREFACE

Our experiences make us who we are. Our genetic matrix provides structure; however, the environment feeds the behavior whether good or bad. The process of building our personalities and traits starts when our hearts begin to beat. Many of us are treated lovingly as infants and children, while some of us are neglected and abused. Some of this negative treatment is so subtle that most of us would never think of it as neglect or abuse.

Abused children appear normal, but tend to act out learned counter-productive behaviors throughout adulthood, and often mistreat their own children as they were mistreated. The abuse, subtle or severe, predicts a traumatic outcome. The resulting neurobiological and behavioral reactions produce diseases that emerge in adulthood.

In the 1990s, the impact of these tragedies motivated me to research ties between unappreciated childhood depression, its origins and its progression to heart attacks when a child becomes an adult. And that's where the original title for this book, *Heart Attacks Begin in Childhood,* a metaphor, was born. Heart attacks are only one example of the health issues that have their beginnings in childhood and this book is about all of them. Though there is much work to be done for the children in need, I chose to focus on "normal" adults with the hope that you, the reader, might influence normal children and other parents, too.

Once a child reaches adulthood, awareness of the conditions and choices for change must occur willingly to avoid the full impact of the developing behaviors and diseases, the storms within. The struggle getting there changes us for the better while further change gives us confidence and hope needed to sustain the effort. Change, when an option through choices, is the essence of prevention that can significantly slow or stop the developing diseases that often cluster together. Choices give opportunity for change, give new freedoms and the chance for growth and independence. Thus, the title: *CHOICES*.

THE POWER OF CHOICE

Life is a sum of all your choices.
—*Albert Camus*

We need to teach the next generation of children from Day One that they are responsible for their lives. Mankind's greatest gift, also its greatest curse, is that we have free choice. We can make our choices built from love or from fear.
—*Elisabeth Kubler-Ross*

It is our choices ... that show what we truly are, far more than our abilities.
—*Anonymous*

Your life is the sum result of all the choices you make, both consciously and unconsciously. If you can control the process of choosing, you can take control of all aspects of your life. You can find the freedom that comes from being in charge of yourself.
—*Robert F. Bennett*

When I make a choice, exactly who's making it? Is it really me or someone else, one of the influential persons in my life who instilled my patterns for decision-making? Have I looked at the facts and my feelings about them or am I choosing instinctively? Do I really know myself as I think I do?

CHOICES

Consider these questions about choices in an outside context, for a moment. Both Joe and Marlene came as patients referred to me.

- Joe is a middle-aged, hard-working traveling business executive. Out-of-town on business, Joe was enjoying a big dinner when without warning he suffered a sudden cardiac arrest. Luckily, one of his colleagues knew CPR. By the time the EMTs arrived, he had responded successfully to the CPR. To everyone's amazement, however, he flatly refused the EMTs' urgent request that he go to the hospital ER. He shrugged them off, insisting he was fine. But over the next ten days, he couldn't muster the energy to work or function as usual, so he came in to see me. After a brief consult and an abnormal electrocardiogram, I sent him right to the lab for a heart catheterization. As I expected, the test confirmed that he had survived a heart attack that had destroyed significant heart muscle. His earlier refusal of treatment right after the attack meant he had missed the opportunity for immediate intervention that would probably have limited damage to the heart. Now as we talked over options to treat the damage and steps he could take to avoid new problems and help recovery, Joe continued to struggle. He threatened to check out of the hospital, waving off any talk about his high blood pressure or other problems we needed to address. Our challenge was to help Joe discover and choose a healthy path to follow. At that moment, however, he wasn't even willing to ask the right questions. What kinds of experiences do you imagine might be driving Joe's denial and self-destructive choices?

- Marlene's attitude seemed very different from Joe's. She was late for the biopsy on the lump in her breast, she explained, because shopping and delivering the groceries for her mom and a sick neighbor took a little longer than she expected. But she laughed and apologized. And on her follow-up visit she brought flowers from her garden to the office staff to make amends. The diagnosis was cancer. "Well, that's a bit scary," she said, "but I'll just go forward. What else can we do?" Marlene's upbeat attitude just after her diagnosis amazed her friends, yet seemed so like her. For the past three years, she had nursed her husband through his final illness with that same quiet positive attitude. She was realistic about the situation but rarely "down." If friends said, "You need to take time for yourself," she'd respond, "Oh, I do. I'm happiest when I can be doing something." So those friends weren't surprised when after her cancer surgery, she was soon back caring for others, even on occasion pushing off her own chemotherapy sessions so she could be there for someone else. Marlene really did seem able to let go pressure and just be in the moment, but they wondered if she perhaps regularly pushed herself too much or neglected her own needs.

What strikes you first about the choices Joe and Marlene are making? Perhaps, how unusual their choices seem to be? Compared to how most of us might respond to these life-changing situations, the responses made by Joe and Marlene seem extreme. Their responses also seem to be opposites. Certainly, they make us consider what kind of experiences and personal history may be behind their unusual choices.

Life is filled with encounters and situations that require hundreds of choices daily. Here too, personal experience shapes the small choices we make constantly. Some choices are conscious; others are automatic responses. All have consequences—some positive, some negative. We may not appreciate the impact of these choices and their consequences, but cumulatively these choices continually shape who we are. Over time, choices shape our bodies and our health. Choices shape our minds and our sense of well-being. Choices shape our sense of self.

Choices shape our relationships. In all human encounters, communication takes place on several levels. There are the words, the message behind the words, and the nonverbal communication of tone and body language. Our choice of response must instantly take all these levels into account. And our answers will affect ourselves and our relationship with the other, whether he or she is a passing acquaintance or someone important to us. These realities apply to the small instances in a normal day and to big, "important" events.

CHOICES

Where Do Our Choices Come From?

Why do you make the choices you do? Why do I choose as I do? We learn our foundational repertoire of behaviors from our families of origin and other significant people that we encountered as babies and children. Many of our basic ways of relating to situations and people go back to these early experiences. This is particularly true if we have never taken time to examine what choices we make and why we make them or where we learned to make them.

As we grow older, we typically experiment with independent behavior and breaking away from family models. If we have particularly wise and self-aware parents, they may help us think through our behaviors and make new or different choices that are appropriate for us. But in most cases, we parents and children muddle along doing the best we can without thinking about why we make the choices we do. We simply live the status quo that we inherited. That means that we recycle the behaviors that we absorbed from our early examples. Some of the behaviors and ways of coping and relating may be excellent; all too often, many are negative because they are no longer relevant or appropriate for our current lives. If we have experienced very stressful or abusive situations, even if they are relatively few, our choices and decision making have probably focused on self-defense and coping.

Choices, Life and Consequences

Life, like an adventure, can be simple or complicated, challenging but fun or harsh and destructive. Life, like a river, flows on whether we're a part of it or not. Life brings change and change is what we respond or react to. We want to be in charge of our lives, not at the mercy of outside events. The goal is to free ourselves from life's many burdens without negatively affecting our health or relationships. We also want reassurance that we can and do act out of our own free-will.

Life doesn't have to be a roller-coaster ride, full of abrupt ups and downs. How we make choices and decisions has a lot to do with whether we set a balanced course or are at the mercy of the roller-coaster influence of outside forces. The process of decision-making can be well thought through and intentional or we can leave it to chance and circumstance.

Making choices on-the-run or instinctually is similar to trying to choose the correct fork in the road after you've already passed it. Unless, through intentional observation, we've become familiar with the territory or have developed an internal compass as a source of consistency, our choices may disadvantage us. If left to chance, our choices might be smart and appropriate or "magical," inappropriate, harmful, or even stupid. Remember, our patterns for decision-making began forming in infancy, shaped by our experiences. The important fact to understand, however, is that we can continually modify these patterns for the better. Developing choices and decision-making skills that benefit us can be a powerful tool for health and happiness.

Life's struggles and health problems don't appear suddenly, but over time. Many typically result from consistent, long-term behaviors, often of our own choosing. Heart attacks and heart disease begin in childhood, for instance. There's no quick-fix for stabilizing or reversing chronic illnesses and diseases, but there is hope for control.

Conflicts in relationships don't typically spring up overnight but are shaped by years of interaction. Additional outside stress can make problems in relationships worse.

For our heath and relationships, for our overall well-being, we need to begin to think through these issues. After all, we aren't required to live in a reactive mode. We have the privilege of using our minds and thinking our way clear.

Just as they did for Joe and Marlene, choices confront us at every step along life's way. Consequences of even our simplest choices influence us more than we know at the time we make them. Many factors help shape each choice. We need to approach choices as if we own them and take responsibility for them and at the same time do our homework to lower the surrounding stresses and to avoid misinformation. In so doing, we better accept the consequences and thus, expand our abilities for making choice. As we continue, we handle choices and decisions more skillfully. We learn when opportunities don't go our way, we can fine-tune our approach for the next challenges. Therein lie the power, strength and hope to continue in the struggle.

What Does This Book Offer You?

A Path to Your Optimal Potential

Today, this week, this year—are you living the rewarding life you envision for yourself and your family? How far have you progressed toward achieving your hopes and dreams?

If we're honest with ourselves, most of us would have to answer, "not really" and "not far enough" to these questions. The routine pressures and duties of daily life keep us running. We struggle to carve out time for ourselves and our families and the things we enjoy together. Coming from all directions, the demands never cease. We cope the best we know how, of course; but too often, we feel that life is out of balance and that we've lost control. The "best we know how" stumbles in the face of relentless challenges. We stress out. Our dreams and visions fade; we settle for "what is" and we pay the price.

Stress in many guises pervades modern life. It relentlessly attacks our health and enjoyment of life. It poisons our relationships. Most of us don't cope well with its insidious pressures. Why not? Because we usually react to stressful situations with coping strategies we learned in childhood—strategies that have become "the best we know how." Rather than choose responses that promote our physical and emotional well-being, we recycle reactionary attitudes and negative behaviors that trigger biological damage and increase feelings of pressure and anxiety. And we don't even know that's what we're doing.

But you can wake up and change for peace and new vitality if you know how to choose to change. This book will show you how to uncover the old, outworn patterns that block progress and learn to let them go. You will also learn techniques that enable you to breakthrough to new responses that defuse stress and free you to be the person you want to be. You can learn how to make new choices that enhance your health, your relationships, and your happiness. You can live fully in the moment, without regretting the past or fearing the future. You can live up to your stars and not down to your labels. You can change and be your best.

The problem

Nobody really likes change. Our built-in independence resists the idea that choosing change may be necessary. It doesn't matter where the change message is coming from either—our doctor, our spouse, a friend, ourselves. Often we may hear the suggestion as a criticism. A negative. Even when we know better.

The solution

Viewing change as an option of choices is a better approach. It's one we can engage and own because there are excellent techniques to help each of us learn for ourselves where the barriers and the opportunities are in any situation and learn how to choose the most effective responses. Guides in this process will be our own values and goals.

Thus, this book *CHOICES* is about you. And if you use *CHOICES* as your personal workbook, under your control, here's what this book can do for you.

- The insights (and exercises) will guide you to an increased awareness of what's happening both within yourself and between you and other people.
- As a result, you will be better able to recognize circumstance, events, and personalities that challenge you.
- You will be better able to understand why you are the way you are and how these realities affect you at work, play and in relationships.
- You'll better understand why you voluntarily—yes, voluntarily—let in unwanted stress and strain.
- You'll learn and practice choosing healthier methods of dealing with and negotiating the stress and adversities of daily life. These methods strengthen your freedom of choice.
- You'll develop understandings and methods that free you from learned entrapments and restore your real freedom to act and be as you truly choose.

CHOICES

Most important, *CHOICES* will open up numerous opportunities for enjoying your life and the relationships you value.

The goal is to help you live life to the fullest day by day. Isn't this what you were born for?

1

First Steps— Waking Up
to the Best You Can Be

In this chapter

An overview of the challenges, the barriers, and the promise of choosing new, positive responses for a happier, healthier, and more meaningful life.

The Challenge: To be at Peace with yourself, to deal with the circumstances facing you, and, at the same time, to be your best for yourself and for those within your personal circle.

The Barriers: Stress, busyness, and worn-out responses.

How is stress affecting your life? It is, whether you are aware of it or not.

Stress—overt and hidden—is:
- attacking your enjoyment of life
- damaging your health
- poisoning your relationships

Ignore it at your peril. Literally. But you can turn the attack back. By listening to the wake-up calls all around you, you can unlock the knowledge within your past experience to breakthrough to *new choices* that will enhance your well-being, your health, and your important relationships.

Do the wake-up calls in any of these stories have a familiar ring?

After hearing the results of his diagnostic tests, Jeb was honestly wondering: "What did I do to deserve a blocked artery? Where did it come from? No one in my family has heart disease. I don't have much stress. I'm a pretty normal guy. I don't smoke and my blood pressure and cholesterol are normal. I love my work—I've been in the same firm for eighteen years and I can pretty much direct my own course. I'm disciplined and good at what I do. In fact, I thrive on the challenge of higher workloads and the buzz that comes from beating the deadlines that go with that territory. I've known others who were stressed, and I'm not like them, uptight and all in a flurry. I really try to be aware of stress and defuse, so what am I missing?

Allison came in hunched over and feeling awful. She complained that her back and chest hurt, especially at night when her chest burned. "My stomach seems to stay upset, and I don't sleep well. Seems like I don't concentrate or remember as well, and I'm only 41. I just feel burnt out—not just my job but on life in general. I guess I'm in good company on the job front—"cause I read somewhere of a poll where 70% of Americans said they felt burnt out in their jobs. Maybe it would be different if the company really used my talents but it seems I do nothing but key things into the computer and crunch numbers. When the day's over I'm too tired to date or go out with girl friends. I do try to get down to see my folks at least once a week, sometimes twice, even though they are sixty miles away but all the thanks I get for doing the little tasks or favors they request is to be put under the microscope. My mother seems to notice every pound I've ever gained or lost. I'm sure ready for a change."

"But I run 10 miles a day . . .and I eat like a rabbit, all green stuff. I've dropped down to ideal weight. What do you mean, I'm missing the boat?" Darryl shouted as he thrust his face, flushing red with anger, toward mine and stabbed a hand wildly in the air. He was a 40-year-old colleague and a successful surgeon. But right then, he looked like a four year old throwing a tantrum. Darryl was more than a little out of control. He wasn't just acting like a four-year-old, at that moment, he was stuck right back in his past, using the same reactive response he'd learned as a pre-schooler. If I were to tell him his heart attack (or the gut-twisting tension in his marriage) had begun in childhood, he'd probably explode. Yet that simple statement would be nothing less than the truth.

Did You Hear Any Echoes of Your Experience in These Stories?

Of course, your life story, like everyone's, is unique. But it's not perfect, is it? The circumstances of modern life tend to produce stress, no matter how good one's coping mechanisms. Health and relationship issues tend to crop up from time to time, too, for everyone. All too often we tend to live down to the labels of our past and not up to the stars of our dreams.

What's going on in your life? It's never too late to wake up to what's happening and choose new responses. You can use your feelings and experiences as cues to lead you to the facts of what's behind negative behaviors and choices. You can make new choices. You can be who you want to be and you can have the life you desire and deserve. You can be your best—the person God intended you to be and that you want to be—but first you have to wake up.

Wake up to what's really going on behind your experiences and feelings:

Wake up to how you may be recycling negative behaviors from the past
. . .Choose awareness

Wake up to what you value
Wake up to who you are and want to be
. . .Choose to respond, rather than to react

Wake up to the labels you've been given
Wake up to your dreams and the promise of a unified life
. . .Choose to live up to your stars,
not down to your labels

Wake up to the power of being yourself at all times
Wake up to the importance of your relationships to really living
.. .Choose to be "you" all the time and everywhere

Wake up to the richness of connectedness
Wake up to the power of spirituality
. . . Choose a greater sense of personal power and control

Wake up to the fact that you can choose to change
to achieve the life you desire and deserve.

You can choose to be your best. This book first offers a wake-up call to help you identify some of the stumbling blocks in your path, particularly those you haven't been able to see. More important, the book then helps you discover how to make the future what you want it to be by rethinking your mindset and making new choices. The insights and techniques shared don't tell you where to go—that's entirely up to you—but I hope they'll provide a map of possible routes and some strategies for choosing the direction that fits you.

Waking Up to What Stress Can Do

We live in high-stress times that challenge us daily. Here are just a few examples.

- We care deeply for our families, but the busyness of our lives pulls each family member in several different directions daily and makes it difficult to connect.

- Rapid changes in the workplace and volatile economic times have increased stress in the workplace—and even more so after a job-loss. National surveys indicate that from 26% to 40% of workers describe their jobs as extremely stressful.

- The continuing threats of global terrorism and war have brought vulnerability and violence frighteningly home to us in the United States.

- Diversity has its benefits, but hatred is on the rise and is somewhat generated from partisan politics and general group differences that contribute to personal stress wherever you stand on particular issues.

- All these stresses and many more rush at us constantly. How we handle these stresses has a direct impact on our physical health and well-being. Scientific research is continually revealing ways in which our attitudes and behaviors affect our biology. This impact in fact, begins at the genetic and cellular level and builds from there.

Most important, however, we can influence how the interaction between stress, biology and behavior affects us. We can learn to use our attitudes and behaviors for our benefit and health—and that of our relationships—or we can be trapped in recycling negative behaviors that ratchet up the risk of chronic diseases such as heart disease, high blood pressure, diabetes, and cancer and wreak havoc with personal relationships. Taking positive action or staying trapped—it's your choice.

Showing you ways to define and make positive choices for your life, health, and aspirations (not somebody else's life or some "typical" life) is my goal in this book.

Choices, Childhood, and Health Problems?
What's the Link?

Nobody chooses to have hypertension, heart disease, cancer, or some other health problem, do they? Of course not. Although most of us may not pay proper attention to the various risk factors for chronic disease, not paying attention to risk factors is far from the whole story. Underlying these risk factors (that tend to emerge in adulthood) are behaviors, choices and habits that are rooted in childhood experiences and shaped by what we learn through our early relationships with people close to us and with our environment. These learned behaviors and choices—what I call our "working model"—shape our ways of relating to people and responding to what happens to us. Our working model also shapes our biology and our health. In fact, we human beings remain works in progress for our whole lives. We continue to develop and change not just physically but also emotionally and spiritually. This book shows you how to tap the power of this dynamic ability.

Nature or Nurture?

Psychologists, biologists and child development specialists have long debated just what roles nature (genetic potentialities) and nurture (environmental interactions) play in shaping an individual's personality and biology. Scientific evidence—as well as common sense—indicate it's both. Each of us is born with a genetic makeup inherited from our parents. Those genes contain many potentialities for various outcomes, including triggers related to various health conditions, such as heart disease or cancer, for instance. That's nature.

Something then must interact with those gene potentials to turn their effects on or off. These potentialities include both protective responses and those that lead to negative consequences. Individual attitudes and actions can help trigger or suppress each potential outcome. That's where nurture—and our individual choices—enter the mix.

Think back a moment to Darryl, the guy who was exploding in my office about his heart troubles. At that angry moment, Darryl was choosing to use a "working model" straight out of his childhood. Combined with his blocked arteries and weakened heart muscle, his reactive, defensive behavior was propelling Darryl toward more heart and health problems, by generating more and more inflammatory changes. In spite of faithfully following his prescribed diet, exercise, and medications, Darryl was not just missing the big picture, he was caustic to the core. His hyper vigilance to the details was controlling his decisions and his life, rather than the reverse. And worst of all, he was unaware and was actively denying it.

Waking Up to the Big Picture

Like Darryl, the way most of us choose to live daily is damaging our health and our relationships with those we love. As a result, these choices are also damaging our happiness and enjoyment of life. That's not too strong a statement. Some of us, of course, know we need to make some changes and are ready. Others, like Darryl, are blind to what we need to do. But achieving a healthy, fulfilling life is something anyone can choose. Choosing to change can make a tremendous difference in your well-being even if you are fighting heart disease, cancer, or another chronic or life-threatening health problem. It can make a big difference if you just wish to prevent such future problems.

What About You and Your Story?

This book's goal is to help you look at your life and wake up to new possibilities. Its strategies and techniques empower you to break-through to a better way of living. The insights and answers you need to achieve your goals are locked inside your personal experiences—your life story. *CHOICES* provides a step-by-step plan to help you:

1. Explore your past to identify and strengthen positive behaviors and to quit recycling negative behaviors that have outlived their value.

2. Discover the freedom to find your true self—the person of value you are—and to think about how you want to grow in the future.

3. Learn how to use your feelings as guides that can point you to the underlying facts of what's really going on in your life and in your important personal relationships.

4. Use these insights to get beyond your defense mecha-nisms and reinforce the changes you decide to make.

5. Create and nurture the positive, life-giving relationships you desire—with spouses, children, parents, friends.

6. Draw on the spiritual aspects of your life for support, strength and positive growth.

7. Recover from or deal effectively with serious physical illnesses and chronic health challenges or disease.

The cutting edge concepts in *CHOICES* blend the research of different sciences and my years of experience as a physician. The goal is to enable you to apply these vital ideas to your individual situation. After all, this is your life. Are you really making the most of it? Ask yourself: What's important, what's significant in life? Is it just about me, or what? When I'm angry and arrogant, do I really know what's best for my family and the course we should plot?

This book is about anxiety, stress, control, anger, isolation, and depression—those ills of modern life—as well as their relationship to other traditional risk factors for chronic diseases (such as lack of physical activity, being overweight, having high cholesterol, having high blood pressure, smoking, having diabetes, etc.) and their effect on your total health and well-being. It's about new ways of making decisions; it's about avoiding making decisions only with our emotions, which hold us hostage to our past. It's about finding the peace of mind that is already inside ourselves if we will only choose to release the too tightly held past. It's about growing through the spiritual power of choice and a closer relationship with your Creator.

Will This Approach Work for You?

At this point, you may be thinking, these are exciting, lofty goals, but will they work for me? Is it really true that simple insights and techniques can enhance not only my physical health but my emotional well-being and the quality of my relationships?

Yes. Absolutely, yes—if you take the time to think through, absorb, experience and act on your choice to change. There is no quick fix. Choose change and begin working on you: it's a process you can do. These concepts and techniques will improve your health, relationships and your total life. And I've seen how powerful they can be in my own life and the life of my family.

In fact, my first insights grew out of my own experience. My father was a successful businessman and civic leader, and he commanded my utmost respect and awe. But he had a quick temper and often expressed it fiercely and used it as a controlling mechanism. I vividly remember telling myself how different I would be as a father one day. (Doesn't that sound familiar?) Then years after leaving home, as a young physician, husband and father, I found myself in stressful situations reacting with anger and causing myself and my family distress. When I looked in the mirror one day, I saw my father: I saw myself reflecting the negative coping behaviors shaped in my childhood. I felt trapped, not in control.

That personal insight together with my patients' pain impelled me to seek sound scientific understandings and practical techniques that could enable individuals to use the powerful connections between mind, body and spirit to breakthrough to new healthful ways of acting and living. In a journey of many years, I have discovered and been able to test with hundreds of individuals how to use powerful, yet simple ways to free one's self from habits of being and acting from the past and move from there to make positive, permanent changes. You can do it, too.

2

Stress—The Neglected Risk Factor for Trouble

How We Handle It Based on Our Working Models

In this chapter

You certainly know that life is filled with stress of all kinds. But do you understand just how your reaction to stress has shaped both your health and the way you relate to people and the world around you? The process starts the day you were born.

This chapter explores the biological and psychological roles stress plays in physical and emotional development. Human responses to various stresses play a role, for instance, in how brain structures develop from infancy onward. When stress collides with the "good" coping strategies learned early in life from caregivers and personal experiences, surprisingly, the outcomes are often "bad" for health and well-being in adulthood.

But choices and change for the better are possible and powerful. Such change starts with understanding what's been happening beneath the surface of personal experience, history, and feelings. The real-life experiences of Eric, Tom, and Mary help frame the discussion and bring the scientific concepts alive. But more important, their individual stories demonstrate that choices and change for the better are possible and powerful.

ERIC

In the middle of the work day, Eric White began to feel as if someone had suddenly lowered a heavy weight onto his chest. He took a deep breath slowly, trying to ease the pressure. But it seemed to increase. Was this what a heart attack felt like? Surely not? Whatever the problem was, Eric was sure he could overcome it, take control, stay in charge—that approach had always worked for him in business and in his personal life.

As the pain increased, he felt a little faint. Maybe he ought to get to a doctor. Call 911? No, he could make it. Hadn't he always managed on his own? He reached his car and headed toward the hospital, fighting to focus on the road, pushing away a rising faintness and anxiety. Pain won the battle. Right in front of the hospital, Eric passed out and crashed into a telephone pole. Arriving almost immediately, the paramedics rushed Eric into the emergency room where the trauma team swung into action to treat what was diagnosed as a major heart attack.

I met Eric hours later in the Intensive Care Unit when I was called in because he was extremely anxious and panicky—how could this be happening to him? Almost shaking with strain and fear, his wife kept vigil at his bedside, struggling to stay positive and "in control" for Eric's sake.

TOM

Not too long after, I was called to the same ICU to counsel Tom. Earlier, he had been rushed to the hospital after being revived from sudden cardiac arrest. The worst part of the experience, he later said, was regaining consciousness in the middle of tubes and wires and a jumble of confusing noises and short bursts of visual images, like scrambled movie clips. He was one angry man. He lashed out against the equipment. He ignored the requests of the ICU staff—particularly that "sassy woman" (the nurse). Who the hell was she? And why should she have any authority over him? Nothing—no reassurance, no request—seemed to dent his stubborn, angry, emotional armor. Finally, his personal physician was able to get him to at least comply with treatment. The fact that he was lucky to be alive and was still in serious danger had not even registered yet—only two percent of individuals who suffer sudden cardiac arrest outside the hospital survive. (Technically, in fact, this event is called sudden cardiac death!)

CHOICES

MARY

Unlike Eric or Tom, Mary wasn't worried about losing control or anything like that, she just didn't want to "be a bother." But after the "little pain" in her neck and arm had gradually worsened over three or four hours in the morning, she called to see if her primary-care physician could work her in "without too much inconvenience." She didn't want to make a fuss. After an initial evaluation, her physician, of course, had her taken directly to the Emergency Department as quickly as possible.

STRESS—The Neglected Health Risk Factor

Eric, Tom and Mary are in the middle of high stress events. No doubt about it—heart attacks qualify as high stress. What they don't know at the moment is that stress and their reaction to it throughout their lives has played a major role in bringing them to the emergency room with heart attacks. Eric, Tom, and Mary aren't unusual. In fact, I've chosen to share their stories because their lives, experiences and attitudes are common.

Most of us are certainly aware that our lives and world are filled with stress of all kinds. But as a cardiologist who specializes in prevention and rehabilitation for persons with heart disease, I know that most of us have very little understanding of just how our reaction to stress in all its many forms has shaped our ways of relating to people and the world around us and shaped our health from the day we were born.

Stress Begins to Affect Health with Choices Made in Childhood

In fact, stress begins laying the foundation for health or disease at the moment of birth when an infant leaves the security of the womb and enters a strange, noisy, confusing, complex environment. Put most simply, potential health consequences start with each individual's reaction to stress. Look carefully at that sentence again. Stress in all its infinite varieties is not the problem—it's how we react to, receive, or handle stress that can help us or hurt us. And that reaction begins with our first days of life. An infant begins life with a specific genetic heritage and potential. With birth itself the infant begins what will be life-long interaction with other individuals and different, specific environments. The first important "choices" are made for every infant by other people.

Stress—It's a Fact of Life and Health

For a moment, imagine yourself as a newborn again. Any new experience is stressful, isn't it? Even for adults. And each day an infant faces dozens of new stimuli. A baby must adjust to being a separate individual, no longer physically connected to the mother. It must learn to eat, adjust to changing sounds, light, dark, images, temperatures, touching, the need to eat, bodily functions, and on and on.

Well, you say, what's so unusual about that scenario? It's just life. That's absolutely right. Stress in its broadest sense is a normal, unavoidable, even necessary condition of life. As one comic said, life without stress is called *death*. Even a lifeless rock experiences stress: As the rock lies on a path, feet tromp upon it, grinding it into the earth. Cycling hot and cold temperatures make it expand and contract, causing cracks. Rainwater seeps into the cracks, freezes in winters and splits the rock. So physical stress exists everywhere for all physical matter in the world.

Compared to a rock, however, human beings are complex entities. We are not just physical beings. We also have a mind, spirit, and emotions. The neural development of our brains, our psychological development and our physical development are complexly, interdependently, and indivisibly woven together. That state makes us human. It also makes possible the development of defensive and compensating responses that can help us cope positively or negatively with the many stresses we encounter every day.

Think again of that newborn baby. How a baby experiences and is helped to receive the new, stressful environments it's encountering—with security or anxiety, with support or isolation, with warmth or indifference, with love or fear—interacts in intricate and complex ways with that baby's ongoing neural and physical development. These experiences also influence long-term health and wellness.

CHOICES

Relationships Are Important to Physical Development

Each of us is born with a unique but inherited genetic makeup. With this "equipment" we begin at birth to encounter specific surrounding environments. Our most important experiences and their memories involve people. People provide relationships. Because human beings are social creatures, we need close relationships to other people starting with our mother, father, and other caregivers to develop not only psychologically and emotionally but also physically. These relationships influence how we react developmentally at all levels to our environment.

Why? As ongoing research is revealing ever more clearly, our physical bodies do not simply house a separate mind and spirit. Instead, right down to the cellular level, biology and psychology are interactive and interdependent. For example, at birth, the part of the brain that controls functions such as breathing or heart beat is completely formed, but the higher brain structures that control functions such as thinking, learning and feeling are still developing. Those higher structures of the brain that control seeing, hearing, language and speech, for example, are also still developing. The nature of our interaction with our caregivers, therefore, affects how we develop physically (starting at the level of how our brain cells are "wired"), intellectually, emotionally, and spiritually. What I call TLC hits, for "tender loving care," are especially important.

Positive interactions and experiences such as touching, holding, and verbal contact make an infant feel secure and foster brain development by nourishing brain "software," its neuron system, and healthful neurochemicals such as serotonin, a substance that helps the body's elements communicate at the cellular level and cope with the potential physical damage of environmental stresses. These healthful reactions work in part by enabling positive gene expressions to take place or by suppressing potentially negative gene expressions.

Lack of positive interaction—too few TLC hits—combined with too many negative experiences make an infant feel insecure, impair neurobiological development, and activate defenses against anything that the infant perceives as a threat. To defend against insecurity, fear, isolation, and feelings of rejection, human beings develop compensations that help them feel okay and in control. For example, crying loudly for an extended period gets attention and care for a baby (or even an adult). These emotional defenses or coping behaviors, however, also cause real physical reactions in the body's chemistry. For example, over a period of years, patterns of anxiety and fear produce chemicals that can damage the lining of the coronary arteries which leads to the buildup and rupture of the fatty deposits that can narrow or block the arteries and cause heart attacks. Such patterns can also produce lethal arrhythmias in the heart.

From an infant's earliest days, then, positive and negative experiences are imprinted in the brain's nuclei, incorporated into the genetically-driven psychological framework, and help shape feelings, thoughts, behaviors and habits, values and skills. Once laid down, these attributes are permanently retained in the neural matrix.

But Are We Permanently Trapped by These Early Experiences?

No. Each individual has many windows of opportunity in life for truly changing his or her working model of behavior, if he or she chooses. But most of us don't think about this possibility often because we don't have the tools to examine what's really behind our customary behaviors and then make deliberate, informed choices for positive or healthful behaviors. We tend to act and react to all life's encounters in ways that our habitual emotional defenses or coping mechanisms inform us feel right or normal.

When we use these emotional defense mechanisms constantly to cope with stresses, they fatigue and overburden our biological protective systems. The overburdened systems may then "stick in the on position," overreact, or otherwise fail, producing physical states that contribute through various pathways to the development of disease.

Among these stresses, for example, scientific research offers strong evidence that certain psychosocial risk factors such as anger and hostility, fear and anxiety, rejection, isolation and depression, and stress in general serve as precursors or triggers for the traditional physical risk factors for heart disease or can activate certain genetic expressions that serve as triggers for these physical risk factors. These same risk factors also lay the groundwork for other health disorders such as high blood pressure, diabetes, lipid disorders (high cholesterol), addictive tendencies (smoking, drugs, alcohol, work, exercise), depression, anger, and anxiety. Many of these conditions open doors to other systemic disorders including cancer, aggressive aging, and lung disease.

Some Real Life Examples of How "Good" Coping Behaviors Can Lead to Health Problems

At this point, you may be wondering exactly what these technical concepts mean in real life. So let's look at how some of these processes led toward health problems for Eric, Tom, and Mary—the individuals whose stories opened this chapter—and how examining their working models for dealing with stress in their lives and relationships helped them achieve better health and well-being.

As I noted at the beginning of the chapter, I'm sharing the stories of these three individuals because their experiences in life have much in common with those of many successful, middle-aged Americans. These are well-adjusted adults, who are partners in enduring marriages and loving parents. They are good at their work. Of course, they have different personalities and the specifics of their personal histories are unique to them, but in the best sense, they are "ordinary" or "average"—just like you and me. We're going to explore how and why they developed their working models for dealing with stress, the effect those working models played in the development of their health problems, and how they were able to begin to adjust their working models to help them deal with these new health challenges.

Eric—An In-Control Over-Achiever

Very early in life Eric learned that he could depend only on himself. He was the oldest of four boys, and his military father was very strict, especially toward him. So as an adult, Eric has felt that his successes are tied to his "toeing the line," crossing all his T's, dotting all his I's, and giving more than 120% effort to every task. He has known better than to depend on anybody. He's convinced he can do and fix anything. He is driven to keep busy. He's in charge and in control.

Where does this behavior come from? Eric is responding as his childhood and later experiences have trained him to do—to work hard to be good enough. Even though as a child and teen, Eric strove to win his parents', particularly his father's, acceptance and approval, his efforts produced only further correction, rarely the praise he longed for.

As an adult, Eric is still using behaviors that originated in his infancy and childhood. When Eric was corrected rather than complimented and encouraged, he acted in ways that would first get his needs met, then would appease and please others. After meeting with failure and rejection, he adjusted to a survival mode. This mode meant that he "should" strive to get the job done with honor—honor to himself and honor to his father's goals, an accomplishment that should earn praise for a job well done. But that praise never came. As a consequence, Eric blocked out his need for praise, buried his emotions under a stoic demeanor, and bought into the belief that he must give near maximal efforts to all tasks, even simple ones. Though this belief gave him no satisfaction, he continually became more driven. If he just tried harder, he felt, maybe the satisfaction he longed for would come at last.

Repeated over time these emotional patterns had a specific, increasing negative effect on Eric's physical body. As Eric processed the events and relationships with his senses and the frontal cortex of his brain, his brain produced stress chemicals which produced physical and emotional responses, which in turn elicited the feelings and biochemical reactions that build memories, morals, judgments, thoughts, more feelings, and actions. In this way, the well-intentioned parenting Eric received unconsciously set the stressful pattern for his way of living and coping.

Of course, like most folks, Eric had many opportunities for change, times when new possibilities seemed desirable and achievable. Two of the most important for Eric were falling in love with his wife and then beginning a new family together. Developing an important new relationship can open a window for transforming the way one person interacts with another so that the relationship is mutually supportive and nurturing rather than becoming another challenging, controlling interaction. Eric, however, did not see this opportunity.

Instead, after marriage, he established a pattern of relating to his wife Anne that reinforced his "in-charge" behavior. He essentially controlled her every move. In turn, Anne provided support that answered his every cue. This pattern of interrelating made both of them vaguely uncomfortable, but at the same time it gave both some sense of positive gain or reward or they would have made some changes through the years.

When it came to his health, Eric felt he was definitely the one in control. His doctor had tried to point out that he had some risk factors for heart disease, but to Eric these seemed too vague and insignificant, too borderline. For example, when Eric had been fighting traffic or battling colleagues in a board meeting, his blood pressure and pulse might shoot up. But he could relax himself, and if the doctor's staff waited long enough, his blood pressure and pulse would fall to normal ranges. The same could be said of his history of elevated cholesterol. Eric tended to ignore his family history of abnormal risk factors such as high cholesterol because his granddad hadn't thought them important and, besides, those relatives had been old when they developed health problems and died. For Eric, health issues, like issues of faith, were things he was too busy to deal with now—he'd think about those when he was older and had met his career goals.

Eric's sudden heart attack dramatically interrupted this daily pattern. At first, after getting over the initial surprise and shock, Eric felt confident that he could take charge and control this heart problem like he had everything else. A positive outlook, a few changes in diet and physical conditioning, and he'd be good as new—right back on track. When his cardiologist recommended that he take a wider view of his needs and consider going to a behavioral support group, he was highly skeptical. But if you pay the man, he thought, you might as well get your money's worth. And he wanted to get back to his best, so he decided to give it a try. His wife Anne agreed to participate with him.

Eric found the process was really difficult, but like everything else he agreed to do, he committed fully to the rehab process. Gradually Eric and Anne began to open up and really look at their individual habits of behavior and the pattern of the relational dance of their marriage. They began to see how they had recycled negative patterns of behavior, which they'd unconsciously learned as children, and to see how these recycled patterns had created innumerable ongoing stresses—both emotional and physical. They began to see how they had also recycled Eric's parents' methods as they raised their own children. This realization was very unsettling. Anne began to acknowledge that she was uncomfortable with Eric's overcontrolling behavior. And both began to realize that Anne's difficult, conflict-filled relationship with Eric's mother had its foundation in the fact that Anne recognized and resented the origin of Eric's behavior when his mom was around.

Eric's most important breakthrough came in a stress management course when he began to keep a chart of his episodes of anger and impatience, both those he suppressed (the majority) and those he verbalized. He began to observe that most had noticeable physical effects that he could feel without medical measurement— his heart beat faster, he literally got "hot under the collar," and his neck felt tight. He started to look behind the rush of anger to find what aspect of the encounter or event was really triggering the feeling, to look for its deeper roots. As Eric looked deeper into himself with his typical courage, he began to see the stress that he was constantly placing on himself and those he loved. Just to take one mundane example, he realized that he took multitasking to an extreme. If he had a twenty-minute trip to a meeting, he'd dictate three letters and make four calls and stop for two errands. Was it any wonder he reached the meeting pushed and impatient?

Beginning with the insights and techniques of the stress management course, Eric began to work to change. When I asked him later what were the biggest benefits he'd gained, he instantly responded, "that I don't have to be right all the time. I don't have to be the alpha male always in charge and so self-focused. And I have let go being competitive in the bad sense."

Eric and Anne have also worked together to shape their relationship into a more mutually supportive partnership. Anne has gradually become her own person, dropping the notion that she couldn't contribute her assessments to decision making, and Eric has worked on listening and responding in ways that aren't controlling. Life has an excitement and new edge for Eric and Anne these days. They realize that they can live more freely without the burdens of old, outworn ways of coping and relating.

CHOICES

Tom—An Intense, Take-Charge Warrior

Tom tended to see life as a battle for survival. If you wanted to reach the top, you had to fight your way up. Tom's father died when he was two, and the story of his relationship with his mother and two older brothers has been one conflict after another—they've fought over everything from "what's the best football team" to family finances. "My way or the highway" summed up Tom's rules of life. In business, Tom has been very successful, though ruthless. And he tended to take the same approach in personal relationships. For example, when a psychiatrist told him that he did not have to let one brother's actions burden him, Tom simply cut off all contact with that brother. Briefly Tom felt satisfied, but his anger at his brother soon resurfaced, even without contact with him.

It seems that Tom has always either controlled or reacted against being controlled, stressful ways of interacting that cost lots of energy. The resulting energy drain caused tremendous wear and tear, raising his blood pressure during and after each encounter. And most every interaction in his life was an "encounter." Previously, Tom had been told that his behavior and intense pursuits might one day kill him. Now his heart attack loomed as death's opening salvo in a war for his life.

Tom entered rehab a miserable and angry man. In a window of sensitivity after his heart attack, he was able to acknowledge the anger that consumed him and realized it was killing him. "I can see," he said, "that I've been sucked into conflict ever since I was a child." He desperately wanted to change. But his working model still presented all challenges as war. So in rehab after his heart attack, Tom threw himself fanatically into exercise and dieting and pursuing change for more optimal health. He has also participated in one type of therapy after another, working towards that change. Unfortunately, Tom's taken the same ruthless, aggressive approach to his rehabilitation that helped get him into trouble in the first place.

In spite of his anger and drive—or perhaps because of them—Tom was forever looking for the therapeutic answers that would truly release him from his many burdens and reduce his risk of heart events. None of these therapies, however, were really helpful until Tom began to see and accept the potential impact of stress, anger and anxiety.

Learning how his ingrained patterns of behavior and emotion create physical stress has proved a real help to Tom in freeing himself from old choices and habits. He's still driven in many ways, but he has begun to see how he needs to let go his anger. He's learning that letting go means forgiving; forgiving his brother and himself and others he's held grudges against. He has even begun to sense the need to forgive his father whose ultimate "rejection" was to die while Tom was young.

As he works through this process, Tom is still learning the power and freedom that forgiving and letting go brings. He now glimpses the reality of being "killed" by his angry, controlling, ruthless behaviors as he has learned about their biological effects. He's working on releasing the fear of the consequences of these behaviors and recognizing that he needs to modify his excessive intensity in his pursuit of better health habits. Tom's still got a long way to go, but he has made a real choice to change and is acting upon that choice.

Mary—Everybody's Rock of Gibraltar

To friends and acquaintances, Mary seemed the ideal wife and mother. She spent her life in giving to her family, to supporting their needs and desires, to being everyone's rock while burying her own needs and desires. Her heart attack came as a surprise. Suddenly, the independent caregiver, everyone's rock, needed support. And where was it going to come from?

Now a widow, Mary couldn't look for help from her husband. Besides she knew it was best that her husband had died first, for starting early in their relationship he had depended on her for nearly everything. Although she had, deep down, resented that responsibility, she had buried those feelings and made the best of it. After he died, she had felt some relief from the emotional burdens of their constant arguments and other demands of their relationship. But she still felt drained of energy. Now, after her heart attack, it took even more energy to maintain herself, and she felt depressed. She admitted to herself that she felt a little hurt that no one was coming to her aid.

Mary's children voiced willingness to help but didn't really come close. Mary knew they were busy and caught up in their own problems and schedules. They were reluctant to interrupt their routines to help her. Although he lived nearby, her son was always too tired, and Mary suspected he was really depressed, too. In addition to living four hundred miles away in another state, her daughter was busy with her children and just not available. Something inside told Mary that they didn't have time for her and really didn't want to help. Mary had always done everything for them and required little responsibility of them. Now that she realized she needed help from somebody, she didn't know where to turn.

With these thoughts in mind, Mary resentfully sought other resources for help. That's what brought her to the support group. For many weeks, she said little in the group sessions but used what she heard to think about her situation. Since she had done so much for her two ungrateful children over the years, she caught herself longing for them to return the love she had shown. She had done so many things for them, freely given them money, sent them on trips. In the midst of one of her many pity parties, Mary suddenly realized that her children were just responding as she had taught them. She had been so organized, so clear about what needed to be done, so quick to do it herself because nobody else did it as well, that she had never asked or even allowed her children to take responsibility. No wonder they were distancing themselves as adults. Even more shocking, she saw that her children had made marriages in which the relational dance mirrored hers and her husband's—one partner doing everything and the other content to be done for.

Many months after her heart attack, when Mary was at last able to talk about these and other hurts in her support group, her first inclination was to call a family meeting to tell everyone just how hurt, angry, and left out she felt. Though such a confrontational approach (but in a different format) might be helpful, she first had to face the fact that holding so tightly to hurts was a way of holding on to her buried anger. She also realized that because of the buried anger, she was avoiding her family and essentially isolating herself. What was best for her and her health was the reverse: to let these hurts go. She also learned that women who become and stay depressed have worse outcomes after a heart attack and that she must accept help, learn new skills and even take medicines her cardiologist recommended if she was to change and enjoy life more. She knew the group was right in telling her she needed to open up, to be more transparent in the group meetings. There was something comforting about this information and her experience of the group. Although she had forced herself to attend at first, the support group had become a safe haven. It was as if the whole experience was giving her newfound freedom. She thought she might even go so far as to say the heart attack was the best thing that ever happened to her because it helped her realize that she had to get out of the controlling environment that she had created for herself.

Mary is now able to enjoy her own life without running or ruining others, for she now better understands the power of a loving relationship and what impact she truly has on her family. She has realized that she can have a greater positive influence on her family with the smallest of changes on her part. She has seen that the children and grandchildren respond with new respect and are now more drawn to her. It's a newfound joy to watch changes unfold and just enjoy her family. She is beginning to re-enter the lives of her children with a true generosity and love without confrontation, for she is free of much of her anger and anxiety and many of her life's burdens. Her goal now is to learn more about herself, to help others understand her experiences (when they are ready to listen), to let go of problems, and to practice healthier habits and behaviors as she pursues her heart healthy lifestyle.

What Eric, Tom, and Mary Have to Teach Us

There's something basic to each of these stories. Many of us can no doubt see some aspect of ourselves in aspects of these three. At the most fundamental level, of course, we all begin with our inherited brainpower and traits contributed from the many individuals in our family tree. Researchers in human psychology have helped us understand that we see ourselves through the eyes and treatment of others: especially our mothers, fathers and other caregivers. Through these experiences we adapt a working model for relationships that we use for the rest of our lives. Many of these experiences are positive because our care is given with love and warmth, making us feel secure. Some patterns of care, however, produce hurts and rejection causing us to protect ourselves with appropriate defenses. As we grow older, we approach relationships with perceptions that may reinforce our responses or we set up situations in these relationships that match what we've experienced earlier and thus reinforce the responses.

A prism for viewing life. We have essentially chosen (without knowing we've made a choice) to see the world of relationships from one view. Ignorant of other possible views, our brains amplify our perceptions, memories, biochemistry and reactions. The hurts and rejections are followed by anger and an inability to trust others, both cloaked by self isolation and/or pride, and an inability to let go the desire to return the hurt and have revenge. Our adaptation mechanisms usually mute these responses so that they are expressed in more socially acceptable behavior such as sarcasm, cynicism, joking, hyper-competitiveness, overachieving and bossiness, to name just a few. We may well function more than adequately.

It's not about blame or guilt. Most people, of course, will not have all positive or all negative experiences and outcomes as they grow and develop ways of relating to others and of coping with the stresses of the world. Instead, as the famous bell-shaped curve suggests, most of us will land in the middle: we'll have much that is positive in our emotional make-ups but we'll also carry plenty of negative baggage. And before you think that I'm blaming anyone (including parents) for that reality, let me say strongly that I'm not. As I said earlier, I'm simply describing what it means to be human.

And what it means to be human is that we are formed physically, emotionally and mentally by experience. Our specific experiences with our specific biology and psychology create memories, feelings, thoughts and beliefs that form a prism through which we view encounters with other persons and our environment. But when our prisms do not change as needed as we grow, they can become distorted and rigid, trapping us in the past.

So how do we continue to grow and change? How can we reshape our defenses and coping mechanisms so that our health and well-being are nurtured rather than harmed? Those same memories, feelings and emotions that create the prism, also provide the cues and tools that can guide us back to the facts that will free us from recycling negative, harmful behaviors. To use these, we must give ourselves permission to re-evaluate the lessons we've learned and the origins of our working models. When we look clearly and without judgment at the complex tangle of facts, we can begin to learn to make choices based on rational perceptions rather than on emotion. We can learn also how to keep the doors open to relation-ships and to growth—and to discovering our optimal selves. We only have to choose to do so.

Yes, let's not misunderstand—we are always our "selves." Everyone has a foundation of self to build on—something solid and good, no matter how buried. My desire is for us to discover that foundation and to recognize we have choices and the ability to look beyond the armor and shields to choose to be ourselves. We can use our emotions, feelings and intuitions as monitors and guides through the adventures of life. We can learn to use all our resources—intellectual and spiritual—to solve the many problems we encounter. And that adventure, then, will be bounded only by the limits of the universe not the limits of personal fears, armor and inhibitions.

3

A Short History of
Why You Are the Way You Are—How Biology,
Experience, and Behavior Connect

In this chapter

Life comes at a price, yet how do we know what price we pay and when it's due? You, like every baby, were born as a work in progress—physically, mentally, emotionally, spiritually. You remain a work in progress for your whole life. Unless we are aware of all the forces that affect us, we may become more vulnerable than we imagine.

We tend to assume we are in control or at least strong enough to manage. In actuality, our minds and bodies frequently can't distinguish between which response mechanisms put us at risk and which help. And the answer to "helpful or harmful?" varies from person to person.

This chapter explores the gradual development of the human mind, body, emotions, and reactions in order to show a) how important balance in the body's systems is for health and well-being and b) how important individual thoughts, feelings, and behaviors are to achieving that balance.

In the last chapter, we looked at the powerful impact that stress and how we handle it can have on our emotional and physical well-being. In this chapter, I want us to look more closely at how all the factors of experience and feelings connect with what's happening inside our bodies. Understanding some of these basic concepts will provide a foundation for what we'll be doing in the rest of this book.

We Are Works in Progress

At birth, each human being arrives in the world as a work in progress. We remain works in progress for the rest of our lives. As newborns—small, unable to control our arms, legs or any bodily movement, dependent on others for food and protection, competent mostly at crying and sleeping—we obviously have a lot of growing and developing to do.

But who, as a child, has not imagined and longed for the arrival of adulthood—when all that "developing" would be finished, when we'd escape the controlling bonds of others on our lives, when we'd finally claim our independence and come into our own. I certainly entertained those fantasies. How about you? Are you laughing yet? Life's never that simple, is it? Neither is the human body.

Human beings are very complex organisms. Who am I? Who are you? Physical body? Mind? Spirit? Personality? Soul? In actuality, the entity we think of as the *Self* combines all these aspects. The result is at once as elegantly simple and as complex as the double helix of the DNA that determines our existence. Most important, this self—physically, mentally, emotionally—is never "finished." For centuries, many philosophers and theologians have described men and women as always *becoming*. What philosophy and faith have discerned as true of the mental, emotional and spiritual self, science is continually discovering to be true of the physical, biological self—the body. And just as important, all aspects of the Self—the physical, mental, emotional, spiritual—are vitally bound up in each other and each aspect affects the development of the other. The interconnections of the developmental process, as far as research has yet revealed, are fascinating.

The Physical Body and the Self Develop in a Context, Not a Vacuum

For every individual the context for personal growth is made up of relationships with family members and other individual relationships together with ongoing interactions with the surrounding environment. Cumulatively, all the interactions and experiences we undergo from birth and infancy onward have an impact on our physical and emotional development. That impact varies depending on each individual's particular genetic makeup and temperament. Although the specific outcomes of experience are unique for each individual, these early interactions help every child develop an initial working model for how he or she will manage future interactions, even into adulthood.

Development Takes Place over a Long Time

Unlike the mythical Greek goddess Athena who sprang fully grown from the head of her father Zeus, human development usually follows a gradual pattern resembling stair steps with extended plateaus. Growth occurs at different rates for different individuals. Observational studies of newborn nurseries in hospitals show how different the infants are. Some cry, some lie still and seem content, some sleep, while others fidget and squirm. Some are colicky, crying and fussing from gas discomfort. Some appear alert and in charge, aware of all around them. At any rate, it's a fact that all babies are distinctly individual, even if what will be their personality or temperament doesn't take more definitive shape until a little later.

Early Development Shapes the Body and the Mind, Forming Patterns for Living

Infants are highly *plastic*. In developmental jargon, being plastic means that important parts of their brains, just like their physical bodies, are not fully developed at birth and need more work. Because the brain is still developing, being plastic in this sense means remaining shapable, malleable, or moldable. Most of the still developing areas involve higher brain functions that control physical and emotional perception and responses, including learning and memory. If these many areas of the brain are nurtured appropriately, they develop fully. If for some reason an area is not adequately nurtured, it won't develop fully, and may even wither away.

The development of the eyes, for example, is completed only after birth through the action of seeing. In the first few weeks of life, an infant's field of vision is fuzzy and fairly narrow (tunnel vision).

The light that enters the eyes signals the brain to continue developing the structures of the eye, brain and connecting nerves that enable normal, clear vision. If something interferes with that process (say the infant were kept in a dark room for the first few months of life), then its vision would never develop properly.

In their book, *Meaningful Differences in the Everyday Experience of Young American Children,* Betty Hart & Todd R. Risley share the findings of their extensive research project into an aspect of how children acquire language and how that's related to future intellectual and academic achievement. Although almost all children by age 2 begin to learn and accumulate a store of words, a vocabulary, even among children who begin to talk at the same time, some children learn words faster and learn more words than others. The authors' research project asked *why*?

The project observed children weekly. All came from stable homes in which the children were loved and well-cared for. When other variables were controlled for, the research concluded that children whose vocabulary grew fastest were those whose parents or families talked to their children more frequently, saying more words to them, engaging them conversationally in the task at hand (eating a meal, washing, looking at something out the window) and responding to their verbal efforts. These children heard more words and learned more words. This richer texture of language appeared to give the children a learning foundation that continued to help them learn more things more quickly when they later went to preschool, kindergarten and/or school. The authors also concluded that establishing such a strong base for learning was pegged to the early years and could not be fully compensated for by more intensive work later in childhood.

These two examples illustrate the continuing process of brain development, both the physical structures and the neural "software" that enable various systems to function.

Though most of this necessary brain development takes place in the first years of life, the brain continues to develop in important ways through adolescence and into adulthood. Even in adulthood, the brain, we are learning, remains plastic in many ways. We continue to adjust the "hardware" and refine or even reprogram the "software" when certain demands are made on the brain, either by involuntary circumstance (such as a stroke) or by choice. That's certainly encouraging news for adults who want to revitalize health, rehabilitate after health problems, or create more satisfying lives and relationships. But back to biology. . . .

Interacting with the Total Environment Shapes The Plastic Brain

With a specific genetic heritage and a brand new body, an infant at birth begins to interact continually with its surrounding environment. Those surroundings are suddenly much larger and more complex than the cozy womb. The world is filled with lights, sounds, lots of movement, eating, breathing, and people—lots of people—touching, holding, talking, cleaning, cradling, feeding, comforting, nurturing, and normally only sometimes frightening or hurting. Received through the senses, these experiences are transmitted to the brain where the chemical and electrical stimuli help shape the physical structures of the brain and the behaviors—both physical and mental—that are controlled by the brain. The quality, number, and nature of interactions play a role in how these structures and behaviors are shaped.

It really is all in your head—the brain shapes behavior. To quote from a standard textbook on neural science, "all behavior is the result of brain function." Dr. Eric R. Kandel and colleagues also state, "Behavior is the result of the interaction between genes and the environment." And what is behavior? Technically the term describes every aspect of human activity, including physical action, mental perception and response, learning, memory, thinking, feeling—voluntary and involuntary. We might sum up behavior by saying, to *be* is to *behave.*

So beginning with birth and using every physical sense, every infant constantly interacts with the people and environment around it. In a complex process, the nature, quality and quantity of those many interactions shape the structures of the brain which in turn help shape physical and mental development and patterns of behavior.

Emotions, the physical manifestations of emotion, and the memory of emotion are important behaviors shaped during this early brain development. Emotions are natural, critical aspects of being alive. Research scientist Antonio Damasso of the University of Iowa says, "Think of the body as the theater of the emotions. . . . Something happens that triggers the bodily responses, and these responses (blushing, a raised angry voice, etc.) characterize the different emotions. But then a second, very important process must take place. The emotion must be mentally assimilated and represented. This involves an entirely different set of brain structures that help maintain the impact of the original emotion.

Why is that important? Because you will be able to use your feelings for future planning, anticipation and decision-making. It will also enable you to empathize with people experiencing the same feelings." As we'll see a little later, all these aspects of emotion play an important role in the complex physical mechanisms that help determine health or disease.

As the newborn sleeps, eats, cries, and interacts, its brain is absorbing, observing and growing. Every waking moment, as the infant receives data, learning goes on. At the molecular and cellular levels the brain communicates within itself using neurotransmitters; messages are sent throughout the body using the nervous system as well as hormones released in the bloodstream. Received from the five senses, incoming data are screened, identified, then sent to the proper structure in the brain—the master control and memory center. The brain responds by adding or dropping neurons, by building new connections between neurons, and so on. The goal is stronger, better function, whatever the task.

Newborns also begin to learn patterns of behavior that depend on memory. Sleeping and feeding schedules, for example, take shape as the baby learns from its caregivers what activities tend to happen when. In the baby's brain thousands of sensations produced by varied activities pass through memory assessment where the experience data are tagged.

Each tag forms a single unit of all the data or facts about a specific experience including the physical and emotional reactions. Tags may allow similar data to be grouped or cross-related. The tag may also signal how long to retain the accumulated data attached to the specific event. Data about some events don't deserve retention, others receive a short retention time and still others a longer time. For example, seeing a leaf drifting down before a window may not be retained as a memory for an infant viewer watching from his crib. But what if a frightening event occurs simultaneously with the experience, let's say a loud clap of thunder occurs and water blows in the open window on the baby just as he sees the drifting leaf. All three events may then be tagged with a higher, more negative (because scary, and therefore stressful) memory code.

At some point, partially genetically determined, the data about any event or type of event become a memory. The degree of positive or negative feeling attached to the memory along with the event's significance for survival determine how much in the fore-front of the mind a specific memory is placed. In my rather extreme example of the drenched baby and drifting leaf, the traumatic nature of the event would probably give that memory a higher retention tag, so that later in life that child might feel uneasy when he spotted drifting leaves. For me, in fact, drifting leaves in autumn always evoke sadness because I associate them with being sick in bed— again a memory tag I can trace to childhood experience.

At a more everyday level, researchers in neonatal neural development theorize that infants develop their first memories as they interact with their closest caregivers. Cumulatively these inter-actions teach them about their "self." For example, the infant brain probably first records verbal and eye contacts and touching, then the absence or presence and timing of contacts with these important individuals. The infant also absorbs the tone (warm, loving, cool, impatient). Just as a calculator clicks away receiving and totaling all the numbers keyed into it, so the infant brain receives and processes every last scrap of experience, and uses them collectively to shape both body and mind, biology and personality, and ulti-mately a sense of self. If healthy infants experience lots of touching and comforting while being cuddled securely and enjoy immediate attention to urgent needs like food and dry clothes, for example, they typically seem happier or more content than infants who experi-ence physical isolation and slowness to respond to urgent needs.

Stress is one of the important factors that helps shape the brain. As discussed earlier, experiencing one's environment and relationships is naturally stressful. That means that from birth onward stress is one of those elements associated with experience that the brain is tagging, accessing, then deleting or remembering and using to shape body and psyche. Positive experiences (those that produce pleasure, security, joy) help to shape healthful behaviors at both biological and emotional levels. Negative experiences (those that produce fear, pain, hurt) help to shape coping, compensating behaviors that were designed to be protective and helpful in the short-term.

But if, for various reasons, such protective stress responses get stuck in the "on position" for too long, the resulting overload can be damaging. As a behavioral example, think of nursing and thumb sucking. Nursing is secure and comforting because baby is being held securely and cherished while an urgent need (food!) is being met. Security and sucking get linked in the baby's mind. So when some later event (not necessary scary, maybe just unknown) makes the baby uneasy or frightened, plop!—into the mouth goes the thumb. With appropriate nurturing, the young child gradually gains a wider understanding of the world and adopts different coping mechanisms and the thumb sucking slips into disuse. Without appropriate nurturing, a child may prolong thumb sucking until it becomes a signal of a certain kind of distress.

Starting as infants, each of us develops patterns for relating to and coping with the people and world around us. Because we learn in response to what we experience, we typically absorb the patterns of behavior modeled by our caregivers, usually our family of origin. This pattern holds true for all types of behaviors including gestures and expressions that are associated with negative physical affects on your health and body.

What kind of reactions and mechanisms does stress trigger in the brain? As stress is experienced, each individual imprints the memory and associated emotion(s), tagging them to biological, chemical reactions. With future encounters, the brain may interpret a new experience as if it were the same as the previous one and trigger the same set of reactions. This *response state* if repeated over and over may harden into a personal *response trait*. Because we model our individual response patterns after those we see most often, many responses may be recognizable as family traits.

CHOICES

What potential effect do these response traits have on physical health? The complex regulatory systems of brain and body exist to maintain a healthful balance. At birth, a healthy infant's body has normal structures in ideal conditions. For every important biological system, such as the heart and cardiovascular system, the healthy newborn's nervous system maintains normalcy within set boundaries for each measure of health, such as blood pressure, pulse rate, blood sugar and the like. Specialized sensors continuously monitor and regulate these elements to ensure proper function. The same process occurs for other systems—endocrine, immune, digestive, etc.

When everything is humming along in perfect balance, in an ideal environment, the body ideally achieves (and maintains) a steady state, an ideal state of balance called *homeostasis*. But no one, not even our newborn infant, lives in an ideal world (at least, not for long). Something is always happening, and those happenings rev up the stress response system.

All responses to stress (such a fear or anger and everything in between) are accompanied by specific neurochemical, biochemical, physical and behavioral responses. Because human biology evolved these responses as defenses for the short term, they typically pose little danger to the body if they occur intermittently and only for short bursts. But prolonged stress creates huge burdens for the body to bear because the defensive responses push the biological systems (and probably the psychological systems) close to their maximum limits.

For example, imagine that you are on a two-lane highway, enjoying your drive through the countryside until you draw up behind a large, slow-moving pulpwood truck. You edge out to pass—the road ahead looks clear. You touch the accelerator and swing out. Just about the time you are midway through the passing maneuver an oncoming car pops up out of an unseen dip in the road. You've gone too far to brake and drop back in; you gun the engine up into the red zone and just nip in front. Whew, close one! You and your car can take that occasionally but would you drive with your car in the red zone? No. You'd soon blow out the engine. You can't continuously drive your body in the red zone without damaging it, either.

The real world is full of ups and downs. Life has pleasures and satisfactions but also lots of hurts, fears and other negative stresses. In response to this reality, medical neuroendocrinologists, especially Dr. B.S. McEwen, have argued that the body maintains balance not as an ideal steady state (*homeostasis*) but by using a variety of adaptive systems that are activated by the nervous system and stress hormone system and that can be used in different combinations to maintain balance. This behavioral model called *allostasis* recognizes that the body has many ways to attempt to maintain an appropriate balance. McEwen has likened the process to the regulation of temperature in your home. The home has a thermostat, heat and air conditioning, and windows and doors. The thermostat keeps an eye on the overall goal. You have several ways to regulate the temp. Put on the AC or the heat? Open windows? Run the fan? Knock a hole in the wall? You get the idea.

When any system must respond repeatedly or continuously to certain perceived stresses, system overload or breakdown may result. The cumulative biological burden that repetitive or continuous work exerts on the body is called *allostatic load.*

How Protective Stress Responses Can Damage the Body

Intensive research in neurobiology and cognitive psychology is leading to a greater understanding of how originally protective stress responses may lead to eventual physical damage to various body systems. The hormones that signal how to handle stress in the short-term and rev up the cardiovascular system and immune system (among other systems) to face stressful challenges begin to damage these systems when they are used so repeatedly or continuously that the alert systems get stuck in the "on" position. Running continuously, the stress response systems trigger injury and inflammation that may be precursors to the development of a variety of disease conditions.

Because our emotions have biological triggers and consequences, feelings and perceptions alone (no matter the event) may often trigger the stress response system. As I noted a little earlier, each response to experience elicits a chemical reaction and lays down a memory of that event in the brain. Repeating that process frequently produces a pattern. After a while, the protective response mechanism may not shut down as quickly after the stressful event ends and eventually may not shut down at all. Throw in a few genetic potentialities (bad or good) that may be triggered by the reactions, and the picture begins to add up to an increased risk for heart disease, cancer or other conditions. If you'd like to see how this process works in more detail, check out the sidebar on the development of heart disease at the end of this chapter.

So, Stress Is, Simultaneously, Both Good and Not So Good

On the one hand, stress is a warning nudge, causing us to move, to look, listen and be more vigilant for possible danger. On the other hand, if we have been repeatedly exposed to negative hits, the stress triggers physical reactions that can be overused. In the 21st century western world, most of us no longer must battle for literal survival, but our alarm systems and internal preparedness still respond as if we had to. The genetic instincts are there fueled by the frustrations of the day and based on past and present hurts and pains. Not only does the alert signal tend to stick in the "on" position, but the stuck reaction takes a toll on the body (though we are usually unaware of this). To these instincts and learned patterns of behavior, we often add anger, which grows with frustration. The result is often cascading bad choices.

What's Turned "On" Can Be Turned "Off"

You are stuck with your particularly genetic heritage, and that includes the biological basis and triggers for your stress response systems. But we are not stuck with our inherited behavioral working models for understanding and managing stress. The basic premise of this book is that we can choose to change. By understanding how our behaviors—emotional and physical—shape our biology, we can identify where the unhealthy behaviors are coming from and choose to change them.

We Are Our Pasts Unless We Choose to Change

As our first teachers, our parents model vital skills for living with other people and surviving in the world. Parents really work at raising us. The only set of directions they have is the patterns (often unexamined) that their teachers taught them. So when I talk about examining your past, I'm not talking about blaming parents. Instead, I'm talking about understanding them and being okay with what was their best. Now it's up to you.

You need to learn to listen to yourself, to listen for the voices that shape your current behaviors. Where do they come from? Which are your childhood voices? Whose voices are they? What messages were you hearing in the past? What messages are you hearing now? What are the real messages about you? Which have you consciously examined and reaffirmed as positive? Which should you reassess today?

We remain limited in our repertoire of how we relate to ourselves and to others until we decide to change the patterns. If our basic pattern is to become anxious then push away during an encounter, we may then rethink the issues and re-approach the other person positively rather than retreat. If we tend to grow angry and strike out, we can re-evaluate and change that approach. By exploring the past in depth, we can eventually understand the original validity of our choices and the fact that they are no longer the right responses for our needs today. Because we were born with the gift of physical, mental and spiritual plasticity, we can put that gift to work for us now. By choosing new behaviors we can often even begin to change and improve our biology.

Only by understanding ourselves in context can we shed the negative burdens of our past, lower the guarding walls, and open the doors to see the positive aspects of our lives. Then we'll free ourselves to see a new hopeful, fulfilling future before us. We will have found a new freedom. We can live more meaningful lives unshackled from our pasts and unload the baggage we haul around. We can free ourselves from many burdens contributing to illnesses and disability. In the next chapter we will explore how you can use your feelings as guides to the facts behind your experiences and relationships.

HOW HEART DISEASE DEVELOPS
An Example of How Body, Stress, and Behavior Connect

Imagine, for a moment, that you are viewing an old black-and-white film clip of a bustling New York City street in the 1920s. The street overflows with hurrying vehicles of all sorts; throngs of people, moving with hurried purpose, crowd the sidewalks. Lining the sidewalks are stores, businesses, and vendors. As the millions bustle up and down the street, hundreds of people turn into and come out of the doors of the various storefronts. The film is moving at such a frantic pace that the scene resembles a stirred up ant bed.

It's not hard to visualize and understand that hectic scene, is it? At a basic level, the activity in that scene closely parallels what's happening daily in the body's blood vessels. If you can picture this familiar scene, you can just as easily understand the basic biology needed to describe what coronary artery disease (CAD) is and how and why it develops in our bodies.

Because understanding these basic concepts can help you understand why making certain choices can make the difference to your health and happiness, don't be put off by bad memories of high school biology or an aversion to blood. Our tour of the remarkable world of the coronary artery and the cardiovascular system and how heart disease develops will be painless. We'll use our image of the bustling New York street to help.

Like a big city, the human body has lots of components and lots of interrelated systems. The basic components of the cardiovascular system include the heart, blood vessels (arteries and veins), and blood. The cardiovascular system is also linked to the nervous system and hormonal system. As we talk about how heart disease gets started, we are most concerned with the coronary (and other) arteries because that's where the trouble starts. Let's take a quick look at a healthy artery and how it works. Then we'll look at how the process of heart disease begins.

A snapshot of a healthy artery

Like city streets, the body's blood vessels are the conduits through which the blood carries oxygen and nutrients to every living cell in the body and takes away carbon dioxide and waste matter. Although an artery looks like a simple tube to the naked eye, it has a number of distinct components. Take a look briefly at figure 1 which illustrates the cross section of a healthy artery.

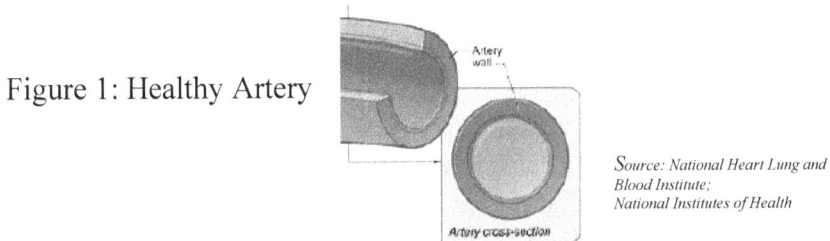

Figure 1: Healthy Artery

Artery wall

Artery cross-section

Source: National Heart Lung and Blood Institute; National Institutes of Health

Observe first that the arterial wall has three distinct layers, each of which has a different function. The outside layers, for example, are composed primarily of muscle and elastic cells that enable the arteries to move elastically, similar to contracting and expanding in concert with the beating heart, an action that may help the heart pump blood throughout the body. These muscular layers of elastic fibers and collagen fibers provide added flexibility and support. Nerves interface with these layers too. The innermost layer forms the passageway (*lumen*) through which the blood flows. This inside wall of the artery is lined with special cells, called *endothelial cells*, that interface with the blood. The artery walls are also designed so that oxygen, nutrients, and other substances that have the right "key" can pass to and from cells in the artery walls and the whole body as necessary just as the people in our street scene pass in and out of the stores and businesses. Because they are so important they are fast-healing (a benefit that paradoxically also opens the first doors to disease).

Flowing through these arteries is blood, a liquid that has many constituent parts. A clear fluid called *plasma* provides a medium in which various substances travel to and from cells. These substances include red blood cells carrying oxygen, disease-fighting white blood cells, platelets and other clotting factors, various lipoproteins (such as "bad" LDL cholesterol , "good" HDL cholesterol, triglycerides, etc), growth factors, macrophages, and so on.

The artery in motion

Now, let's crank up the projector and put all these parts in motion. Remember our street scene—all sorts of people and vehicles are racing up and down the street and in and out of the buildings. In more complex fashion, that's what is happening in your arteries.

There is nothing static in the cardiovascular system. As the body's engine, the heart pumps blood through the arteries to every cell in the body where it delivers nutrients and oxygen and takes away wastes. The blood then returns via the veins to the heart, where it is pumped to the lungs to dump carbon dioxide and pick up a fresh load of oxygen. All along the way the various cells that make up the blood are interacting in numerous ways with the blood vessel walls to do their many jobs, which include feeding, waste disposal, cell maintenance, disease fighting and—important to our understanding of heart disease—damage control.

Damage control is important because all the work of keeping every cell in the body alive and in good health is stressful work. The arteries are constantly expanding and contracting as the pumping heart moves the blood through their channels. Various cells and other particles are passing in and out of cells. Just as the traffic of vehicles and pedestrians causes normal wear to the street and buildings in our film, so the regular work and activity of the cardiovascular system damages or wears various parts. So the body provides protective and healing components whose job is to repair this normal damage, just as a city and businesses might provide maintenance workers. Body and city alike also provide "construction" workers to build new or replacement structures as needed. The overall aim is to keep everything in balance and functioning well. In the body, this state of balance is called *homeostasis*. Ideally, we could sustain our bodies perpetually in this perfect balance. But as the bumper sticker says, "Life happens."

How the trouble begins

But let's suppose for a moment, that a gang of thieves decides to pull off a major robbery in the middle of our street. As they race up to the target in their getaway vehicles, they sideswipe passersby and break down the door of the store. At this point, the police and EMTs, who have been mostly behind the scenes until needed, rush out to try to stop the thieves and care for the injured. The same happens if there's a fire. And the greater the problem, the greater the rescue forces dispatched.

The same thing happens in the cardiovascular system. Major alarms such as damage to the artery lining or a clot or a viral infection such as a cold call forth major protective agents, which go to work until the damage is repaired and healed or the virus is under control.

It's pretty exciting to watch the city's and body's defensive forces kick into action to deal with these major threats. But as we know, major threats are not the norm. Instead, what most affects the quality of life in our imaginary city is the day-in-and-day-out quality of life on the street. Are potholes constantly developing? Do cracks keep appearing in the sidewalks? Just how sturdy and durable are the basic structures? Is the air always smoggy? Do heavy traffic and blaring horns fill the air with noise? How many merchants and business people inside the buildings care just about the quick buck and not the customer? Are growing numbers of pickpockets and purse-snatchers making the street a more dangerous place to visit? Are the stores beginning to look run down? When such negative activity starts happening all at once and keeps progressing, can even the most strenuous efforts of the maintenance, construction and help and rescue personnel restore normalcy? At what point is the whole system totally overwhelmed?

While we can't carry this analogy between busy city streets and the coronary arteries too far, I think you begin to see the basic point that relates to how healthy arteries begin to develop the precursors (or pre-risks) for heart disease. The body's cardiovascular system is set up to work in balance and to deal with normal wear and tear. However, a number of factors (most of which stem from behavior and choice and some of which may be genetically driven) can disturb that balance and overload the system leading to a number of precursors, also called *pre-risks*, for heart disease (and other health problems). In medicine we often call these negative factors *burdens*—because they represent a negative "load" that the body must physically accommodate.

Just as the quality of life on our city street deteriorates as more problems arise, so the more burdens a body's owner or outside circumstances introduce into the system the more stressful that work is and the more damage occurs. The trouble that we call heart disease starts with attempts to control that damage. Warning flags of that trouble often start as early as ten years of age.

To better understand what we're talking about let's zoom in for a close up of how the disease process starts at the active interface between a coronary artery and the blood. Although this process builds over many years, I'll be collapsing the action so we can follow it more clearly. Also remember, that because scientific research is daily revealing more and more about the intricate complexities of the body, this scenario reflects our best understanding at the moment.

How coronary artery disease develops

During every second of life, heart, blood vessels and blood are constantly active and interactive. The heart beats, the arteries pulse, blow flows around and around. At an average heart rate of 72 beats per minute, the heart at rest pumps about 1800 gallons of blood every 24 hours. As the blood flows through the cardiovascular system various events (everything from a high fat meal to the body's chemical reaction to stress to untreated high blood pressure) cause microscopic damage to the special cells lining the inside walls of the arteries. Responding to stress, the brain kicks into action. The hypothalamus produces the chemical CRH which signals the pituitary to produce cortisol and norepinephrine - a neurotransmitter, one of the hormones (with dopamine and serotonin) important for brain function. Cortisol boosts blood sugar for energy and norepinephrine/epinephrine signals the brain and muscles (including the heart) to get ready for dealing with what's ahead. All systems go on high alert—warning, warning!

At the first sign of damage to the inner lining of the arterial blood vessels from any of these causes, the blood's protective constituents spring into action, rushing all the "healers" to the site of the injury, the process of inflammation. But the injury has left the vessel vulnerable because its "stunning" effect has inhibited the protective "juices" (such as nitrous oxide, a vasodilating chemical) that maintain the normal vessel wall integrity. Therefore, when low density cholesterol (LDL-C) arrives—cholesterols are major building blocks for all cells in the body—it is able to enter the damaged artery wall cells. As the tissues react to the injury with this inflammatory response, the other injury fighters (such as platelets, growth factors, and macrophages) also jump into the fray trying to restore the injury.

When certain factors are present, such efforts at restoration can run wild. The result is that cholesterol-rich deposits called plaques begin to develop in artery walls. If this process just happens occasionally the vessels recover, but when the process is prolonged by continual stress in daily life, the switch sticks on and damage to the artery linings continues to build. Over many years, if not controlled, this run-away restoration process leads to the development of vulnerable plaque, whether small or large. Eventually, a rupture may cause a clot that blocks a coronary artery, producing a heart attack.

How does this biological process work in real life?

Let's bring this process down to an everyday level by looking at what happens to the arteries if we engage in three common activities: eating an all-American meal of hamburger and fries, smoking two cigarettes, or experiencing an argument at work.

First, the fat in the meal, nicotine in the cigarettes, and mental stress from the argument can *each* by themselves stun the arterial inner lining, rendering it unable to perform its usual functions and slowing the damage repair teams for as much as four hours. The individual quantities of fat (cholesterol-LDL type), nicotine and stress also cause damaging chemical reactions that produce destructive free-radicals (biochemical products of oxidation reactions) at just the time the protective resources are slowed. Now take these simple acts and multiply them many times over and you see how easy it can be to exceed the limits where the body can protect itself.

Imagine this process recurring many times during the course of the day, maybe thousands to possibly millions of times. No wonder plaquing often occurs at multiple points of higher wall stress, such as at branch-points of the arteries. As more and more abnormal responses are initiated, opposing clean up and restoration processes are not always able to keep up with damage control to counteract the destructive activity.

Over time these behaviors trigger additional risk factors. For instance, insulin resistance and elevated blood sugar come from chronic cortisol elevation (part of the chronic stress response). The cortisol influences the immune system and also can stimulate the cellular structures, platelets and white blood corpuscles. Elevated blood sugars often lead to diabetes, a risk marker for coronary heart disease. Stress-induced increased cortisol may also alter immunity to the point that rheumatoid arthritis or certain cancers may become manifest, depending on genetic and other predispositions.

Genes exert their influence everywhere, at every stage. So do other risk factors such as hypertension (high blood pressure), elevated cholesterol (high total cholesterol [TC], high low density cholesterol [LDL-C] and low high density cholesterol [HDL-C]), and elevation of another blood fat: triglycerides, plus smoking and mental or psychological stress are also significant causes of injury (with more inflammation) to the artery walls.

To summarize then, the disease development is clear: abuse the vessels and they'll respond with change. Change, a natural, compensating, remodeling phenomenon does not know when and where to stop as long as the stimulus persists. The over-compensating processes continue to recruit inflammatory cells to destroy the invading enemy, remove debris and restore normalcy. These protective processes work until they are overcome by the amount of repair needed and then fail to stop the plaque thickening. It may help to liken the momentum of the repair process to the momentum of a train with seven locomotive engines pulling three hundred cars. Pressing the stop button has no immediate effect—it takes miles and miles and plenty of time to stop the beast. It's also important to remember that signs of system distress are present subclinically (that means you can't detect it with ordinary medical tests) many years before visible disease develops. But because each of these negative processes adds to the overwhelmed biological burden, they represent chronic, toxic stress.

Risk factors for heart disease

Heart disease develops, as we can see by now, from not just one cause but a variety of potential causes, which often exist simultaneously. Almost everyone is familiar with the major and other risk factors for heart disease as identified by the American Heart Association and other scientists on the basis of the accumulated evidence of thousands of research studies over many years. The major risk factors include high blood pressure (hypertension), elevated cholesterol (particular LDL cholesterol), smoking, inactivity, and obesity/overweight. Other risk factors include stress (including anger, depression and hostility), and a family history of premature heart disease. We also know that men tend to be vulnerable to heart disease earlier in life than women, but after menopause women catch up quickly. Because the incidence of heart disease is so prevalent in diabetics, it's now called a risk marker, too. As you would guess from the progressive nature of heart disease, the risk of developing it also increases with aging.

Ongoing research is also identifying and studying emerging risk factors such as depression and elevated levels of the chemical called heart-specific C-reactive protein, plus low levels of antioxidants, abnormal blood clotting and high consumption of alcohol. And, I'm sure as research continues we'll discover even more risk factors and pre-risk factors.

The behaviors and choices that shaped your pre-risks and risks for heart disease (and other diseases) started early in life as genetic potentialities, biochemical responses and behaviors that interreact. The good news is that you can examine the patterns of reactivity created by these "choices" and make new choices to change for better health and well-being.

4

Feelings as Cues

How Emotions Can Reveal Facts about Your Experiences and Relationships

In this chapter

What have your feelings got to do with the facts of your life? A lot actually. The emotions and passions that seem to be about current events and relationships also tie you to your past and keep you living there.

In American culture, adults aren't supposed to pay much attention to emotions. As a result hidden emotions may control and trap us into recycling negative or outworn responses and behaviors. But every emotion is a cue that can lead us to discover the roots of those feelings and responses and what values, beliefs, and sense of self they reflect.

Failure to examine the facts behind your feelings practically guarantees that past hurts and fears and old labels will determine present reactions. This chapter not only explains the validity of the feelings/facts connection but discusses important aspects and guidelines for tapping this resource.

My friendship with Dave went back to high school and continued into adulthood. Dave's wife had died the year before, and he had no children. But I hadn't seen Dave in six months when I dreamed about him.

CHOICES

Spotting his car in the driveway as I drove through his neighborhood, I stopped on a whim, thinking he would be home. I found the front door ajar. Knocking on the door two or three times produced no response.

"Hello! ...Is somebody home? ...Dave?...Hello!" No one answered. So I walked in. The place looked a mess. As I went through the front rooms, calling for David, I noticed a large object in the doorway to the kitchen—a huge stone. Was Dave into sculpting? There were no tools nearby. Strangely, I felt a familiar aura when standing near that rock.

Walking through the house, continuing to call out, and finding only silence finally convinced me that he wasn't there. As I turned to leave, I again noticed that large stone slab. It must have been six feet high, two feet wide and one foot thick. What a curiosity. Yet I was drawn to touch it. The surface flaked and crumbled. I touched it again, getting my fingers dusty. Somehow something in the rock connected with me!

So, I began rubbing it and inexplicably singing a song usually reserved for my wife. That strangely seemed the right thing to do. I actually felt a bond with the stupid stone. Then an amazing thing happened. As I rubbed I noticed a sparkle, then discovered metal, then glass: the metal rim of a pair of glasses. As I rubbed more furiously, eyes and a nose appeared .. .

"Dave— is it really you?" He didn't answer. Fear chilled my bones. Was he dead? Had he been killed? Was I in danger? Should I leave? Should I call the police? I pushed away these voices and kept working at the stone. After three hours, I'd uncovered Dave's head and chest. Slowly he awoke and began to speak. The more I rubbed away the stone, the more he shared. It literally took all night to free him. During those hours, Dave poured out his troubles. All his grief, disappointments, hurts, and fears tumbled out. With sarcastic cynicism, he catalogued his anger, burdens, obligations, and expectations from past and present.

I had known Dave was growing more distant and busy, essentially isolating himself. On our last visit, I had found him more cynical than usual. He was having problems in every area of his life, he was tired and frustrated, continually angry, impossible to work with. He had finally piled on so much armor, compensating for all the hurts and accumulated burdens that he had literally turned to stone!

Waking from this vivid, troubling dream, I waited until morning to call Dave. We met for breakfast because he was eager to talk. He shared his distress. He was overloaded with family matters (particularly caring for his parents as the oldest sibling) and pressure from his job (he was unhappy and unfulfilled in his work, not doing what he was impassioned to do, unable to be honest with his boss). Loneliness and grief for his wife just added to the crushing weight. He knew he had mood swings. He was frustrated that everything seemed a bother, and he knew he was too fussy about minor stuff. He felt he was about to blow. He was so tense, he said, that he'd felt chest pressure rather than energy while jogging the week before, though he dismissed that as unimportant.

Alarm bells went off for me. I insisted, against his protests, that he get the chest pain evaluated. Testing confirmed Dave's peril. He ended up with a coronary stent and six new medicines, including one for depression. Though he complains about the number of medicines, Dave's back to his old self, not isolating himself, and more pleasant to be with.

My dream of Dave encased in stone illustrates a message central to this book. We all have the potential to become trapped within an invisible shell of armor that shields us not only from others and our environment but from ourselves. It's layered on year after year and hurt after hurt. What happened to my friend Dave can happen to each of us.

Chapter 3 explained how we develop behaviors and values that mirror those taught us (or unconsciously absorbed) in growing up. In anyone's life, some experiences are positive and others are negative. Unless we look behind the surface of daily life and the accustomed patterns of our relationships, we tend to get stuck. The first step in getting unstuck is to learn what's really going on underneath our assumptions and unexamined behaviors. This chapter looks at how our feelings can lead to the underlying facts about what's positive in our lives and what we need to do to change what's negative.

CHOICES

It's All about Being Your True Self

Though Dave's story is harsh, is any of it familiar to you? Dave's negative behaviors, like ours, often result from a life lived out of the heads of others, ideas and ideals out of the past that fill our heads and affect our hearts and our health.

Life has to be based on and lived from values. Values are the foundation of who you are. Identifying your own core values and separating them from all the other values and voices that assail you is the way to simplify life. Think about it. Instead of wearing so many hats, it's far simpler to be who you are, to be one identity and wear one hat. That way you can perform in all areas of life based on your principles rather than live based on a foundation that you don't believe in. Living somebody else's idea of your life leads to resentment and discontent. These feelings, in turn, can lead to bad choices and unhealthy habits—and thus, to developing risk factors for disease.

Inside each of us is our true self: the worthy person who's lovable, valuable and real. This true self has an identity based on the confidence given by God, a parent, and/or ourselves as mentored by a worthy role-model. But as we live our lives, many of us identify ourselves by our training or title or family role rather than by our core Self. Linking our sense of self primarily to our job and family titles is like eating sugar—your brain likes it but the impact is short-lived and can't sustain the energy needed for a full life. As we cram more activity into our schedules, some of us live as though we're standing in a pot of water with the heat turned on. We don't feel what the gradually increasing heat produced by our single-minded focus is doing to us, both to our health and our relationships, until the "temperature" of stress nears the boil. We may be well-focused for the job, but poorly focused for life with others, unaware and insensitive to those needs, untrained to recognize and change ourselves because of it.

You already hold the key to successful change—your feelings. That's the most important thing I have to tell you in the face of these challenges. Those emotions and passions that seem to be about current events in life also tie you to your past and keep you living there. In the daily course of life and relationships most people tend to take feelings at face value—what you feel is what you feel.

Feelings may be misleading, however, unless you follow them as clues pointing to the facts driving them. You have to delve into your feelings, get beneath them and face them head-on. You are the one to do the work. And it's tough work (not "touchy-feely," fluffy stuff) But you can and will be okay.

Why Feelings Are Important

In our American culture, we adults aren't supposed to pay much attention to our emotions. Instead we are expected to keep them pushed down and invisible—even from ourselves. But ironically, as a result of failing to examine our emotions and what they have to tell us about ourselves, we often act and react to events and other people based on "gut feelings"—hidden emotions that control and trap us into recycling behaviors that hurt our health, not to mention our relationships, peace of mind and quality of life.

Why are feelings so powerful? Feelings or emotions affect our thoughts, beliefs, sense of self, and thus influence our actions, behaviors and lifestyles. These learned behaviors, or habits, and our genetic make-ups in turn determine our health outcomes.

By learning to think of feelings as friends or cues that can lead us to discover the facts behind our behavior, beliefs and sense of self, we can then truly take control to make positive changes that lessen stress and promote physical and emotional health. Taking control defines the difference between reacting and responding. When we react, someone else or some other factor is in control. Without thinking, we give our control away. Responding, in contrast, involves choosing. Choosing gives us space to step back or step aside, to get out of harm's way. This move gives us distance, gives us a chance to collect ourselves, to calm down, and then choose what action or inaction is best. Only then is it a choice.

Feeling anger, for example, does not compel us to act like the stereotypical person who is ranting and raving mad. The same goes for other potentially negative emotions. We can use the feelings as signals that it's time to exert the positive behavior that we desire. It's never too late to take advantage of these powerful insights.

CHOICES

Using Our Feelings as Guides Requires Examining Them Carefully

Many of us assume we've identified our feelings when we say, for instance, "I'm angry" or "I feel good." Yet, we've just skimmed the surface. Anger, for example, is never a primary emotion—some other emotion such as hurt or fear triggers it. And often these triggering emotions follow patterns of behavior that we learned much earlier in life. What was an appropriate response in childhood or adolescence may now be inappropriate in adulthood.

But if we never examine feelings such as anger, frustration, or pride, we'll never discover the primary reason why we feel the way we do. We often recycle negative or inappropriate behaviors that trouble our relationships and present risks to our physical health and emotional well-being.

How? The absence or presence of emotional well-being and peace of mind set the stage for re-enforcing negative or positive "mental videos," images, thoughts and feelings that determine our actions and behaviors. Through these methods, we may mask our true feelings behind the assertion that we actually feel some other emotion.

Dave's Experience Illustrates Hidden Feelings

Look at Dave—he had become cynical, sarcastic, and short-tempered. Little annoyances at work and in daily activities made him see red. Rather than explode, however, he usually just snapped at others or displayed classic chip-on-the-shoulder attitudes. When a prolonged pattern of such behavior meant that co-workers and friends gradually gave him fewer and fewer strokes, he withdrew into a shell of overwork and busyness.

When Dave finally admitted he needed to do something and began to look at what was behind his fog of powerful, if largely unfocused, anger, he began to discover other more primary feelings and facts.

Of course, grief over his wife's death and his great sense of loss and abandonment was an obvious perception. But he was surprised to find when he examined his feelings closely that he was also angry at his wife—how dare she leave him like that. He had depended on her—she was his oasis in a world that piled stress on him. If work frustrations were getting to him, she could help him see the funny side and would soon have him laughing and letting go. When he felt bruised, she'd coddle him until he felt better. Most important, she made him feel good about himself—she liked him just the way he was; she never seemed put off by either his bull-headedness or his I-can-do-it-myself attitudes. By damn, he was mad at God and the universe for so cruelly cutting her life short and for leaving him alone and comfortless.

But Dave's problems with heart disease had begun in his late thirties, well before his wife's illness. Though she'd helped him laugh and relax a bit and provided an oasis when he wanted it, he'd still felt driven to succeed in his work as a marketing executive, particularly by being a good team leader.

I asked him what his leadership style at work reminded him of. He thought a moment before saying, "Well, even as a kid my folks expected me as the eldest to set the example for all the younger kids, to live up to the family expectations."

And what were some of those? Most of Dave's memories emerged as little slogans or attitudes that he felt his parents rein-forced with all the children as key beliefs for successful living:

- keep a tough upper lip
- stand on your own two feet
- be a man
- when the going gets tough, the tough get going
- I'm proud of you for staying in control
- don't let the other guy see you cry

Over the years, Dave had learned to stuff whatever he was feeling down inside so that he lived up to his leadership role, so that he set that example. Even after he reached adulthood, his parents often remembered what a "good" kid he'd been. They'd brag that he'd never needed the attention his younger brothers required or needed rescuing as they had. He'd been a little man right from the start.

How had that made him feel? How did it make him feel even now? A little like the older brother in the story of the Prodigal Son, Dave said—neglected, not given his due, not fully understood, not appreciated for himself, particularly when he'd done all that was asked of him. It wasn't long before Dave began to link his current anger to those earlier feelings and patterns: he'd just lost the one person who did appreciate the vulnerable person he felt inside, who eased his guilt about still feeling vulnerable when it wasn't the "right" or "manly" way to live. No wonder he was finally lashing out at everything. In a sense he was grieving for lost time and lost opportunities, not yet ready to turn to the future.

Our Attitudes about Our Feelings Are Shaped Early

Dave's experience isn't unusual. In childhood, most people are taught to ignore and disregard feelings as unreliable sensations that only expose weaknesses and vulnerabilities. Such teaching is usually not intentional. Instead, it's a byproduct of the way our parents and caregivers handled the bumps and bruises of life (more than the big hurts). Consider what three-year-old Joey is learning.

Out playing one day, Joey tripped and fell, skinning his knee. He couldn't hide the tears and approached his mom for consolation, that special tender love and care that only she could give. Busy raking leaves, she chided him to hush crying, to be her little man and run for a Band-Aid. Automatically, he fetched it to please her and she applied it. Then, to his dismay, she told him to go back to his play without so much as a pat. So he stuffed down his hurt pride that his own mother had not listened empathetically or offered him tenderness.

Although this was not the first time his mother had responded so, it was the first time he noticed feeling upset and resentful for the treatment. Why was that? Perhaps this particular negative "hit" finally maxed out the register in his memory center— that place where positive and negative hits are balanced. (Research suggests that we need 5 positive "hits" to balance 1 negative hit.) As he returned to his play activities, Joey eventually forgot about the incident. But the impact on how Joey deals with his feelings and how he handles and confronts stress will linger. The message? Ignore it, it's not important. Deal with the hurt yourself.

Dave and Joey provide just two examples of how a similar way of dealing with emotion may be learned early. I picked their examples because they are so "normal," because the patterns of their experiences are a part of growing up and nurture for many people. From there, it's easy to think of other patterns that might develop to cope with different stresses, particularly in situations where neglect or abuse exists. To cope with these hurts, it's no wonder that human beings develop *cloaking* emotions such as anger or depression.

How Powerful Cloaking Emotions Emerge
to Cover up the Hurt or Fear

We've seen how Dave's current feelings led back to his roots and how anger emerged in response to his hurts. Because he didn't understand what was going on, he could not let go the past—he just continued to stuff his feelings down until he could no longer contain the anger. Dave's anger was cloaking the deeper, more primary feelings of hurt and fear. Anger is probably the most common cloaking emotion that people experience. And research has convincingly linked elements of anger (particularly the hostility components) to heart disease, Dave's particular health problem. Two other common cloaking emotions are depression and what I'd called false pride or puffed-up pride.

A Window onto What We Know
about Ourselves and Others

In order to grow and choose new ways of responding to daily stress, you will need to be able to look behind the cloaking emotions to discover the underlying feelings and facts. Your eventual goal is to become more open and transparent to yourself first and then to others as you cease to be driven by buried and painful "stuff." I've found that it helps to have a visual window that helps me look at what I'm trying to explore. This tool is called Johari's Window.

JOHARI'S WINDOW	Things I Know	Things I Don't Know
Things They Know	1) Arena - the Open Area	2) The Blind Spot
Things They Don't Know	3) The Hidden Area	4) The Unknown Area

CHOICES

As you look at yourself—in any area—there are things that you know that are also obvious to people who know you. This open window (1) is easy to live in; it's low stress because no defense or covering up is needed. You are yourself and okay with it. But every individual has blind spots (2) things about yourself that you don't know but that others see. You also have hidden areas (3) that are full of feelings and thoughts that you keep hidden from others. Then there is the unknown area (4) which contains the experiences, motivations and stuff that is hidden from both yourself and others, yet these buried forces may be having a profound effect on your behavior.

The goal is to increase the size of the open area (1), to be more transparent to yourself and others by reducing the size and number of your "blind spots" (2) "hidden" areas (3), and "unknown" (4) elements. The goal is to make openness dominant in your life and diminish the stressful power of the other three in your life.

JOHARI'S WINDOW	Things I Know	Things I Don't Know
Things They Know	1) Arena - the Open Area	2) The Blind Spot
Things They Don't Know	3)The Hidden Area	4) The Unknown Area

Using your current feelings as cues to explore the hidden or cloaked facts, to link to forgotten memories and experiences that helped form your current working model, can help you achieve clarity of thought and emotion. This clarity can enable you to affirm good choices and let go negative stuff and refocus on positive new actions. I'll be using this window to help focus your work in this chapter and beyond. To begin, we'll be looking at the areas that contain cloaked and hidden memories and feelings.

Memories Are Tied to and Evoked by Cloaking Emotions

How do negative hits pile up so that they begin to affect biology and behavior? Memories and the memory center of the brain play the key roles. Even when you are unaware of them—which is most of the time in daily life—memories amplify the hurts and hold you to the past.

Let me show you how that works with a couple of examples.

The power of penmanship

When I write out a prescription for a patient or note for friend, I know the bad handwriting jokes are coming. Alas, there's cause—I fit the doctor stereotype for illegibility. Even as it happens for the umpty-thousandth time, I laugh and go along. Inside, I'm seething with irritation; at least I used to seethe until I explored why such a trivial matter should get on my last nerve.

As I looked at the emotions and memories associated with my experiences as a penman, I went back twenty-five years to the time when the hospital and practice with which I was affiliated pointedly asked me to dictate all writing—reports, notes and so on—so that there would be no error. The request filled me with shame. I took pride in my skills as a physician and the request stung like a reprimand.

Looking back even further, I realized that I had rebelled under the discipline of learning cursive. And that rebellion was intertwined with a vague memory of cowering under my angry father's hand as he whipped me for scribbling in an important notebook of his.

Other similar scenes eddied up until they coalesced into a mental image of a spiral of little circles flowing out like a Slinky. Little circles I never would practice enough during class lessons in cursive. Little circles that I still see every time I see a Slinky or a spiraling doodle or even a circular series of clouds. Without knowing it, I had vested such emotion in those circles that to this day they pop instantly to mind anytime I see a flowing spiral.

What did digging up these memories do for me? It let me identify the sense of failure (no matter how seemingly trivial) or lost opportunity that was behind my irritation or anger at being teased about my handwriting. As I linked that emotion with the later shame, I was able to let go the false pride that persisted in linking my handwriting to my medical expertise and therefore was masking the earlier hurt. I then chose a different response—to forgive myself (and my parents) for that early failure to practice and to not "sweat the small stuff."

My experience may be amusing, but it can help us begin to see the roles that feelings and the memories behind them can play in more important and life-shaping behaviors. Vivian's story should make this role even clearer.

Pushing Vivian's buttons

Vivian is a retired teacher who participates in a support group for women who've survived heart attacks. One of her older sisters frequently fusses at her, clearly trying to make her feel guilty. The sister flings out the bait—you are always too busy with your career to take time for family, you ought to take more time for us, you weren't there when Daddy was sick, you never could cook rolls without scorching them. . .and so on and on.

Every time her sister casts out a disparaging remark, Vivian goes for the bait like a hungry trout. Then she feels trapped. "I just want to be free," she says to the group. Free of shame over her sense of failure. Each time her sister pushes the right buttons, she is plagued by the too familiar voices, the messages within her head, telling her what she ought to do and how she's failed to do it. The messages and the feelings they generate are always as fresh as those from her childhood, when this older sister assumed some of the responsibility for caring for the younger children when their mother died. Vivian was not yet in school at the time.

Regrettably, these messages have the same effect now as then—they make Vivian feel defensive, like she's a child again, like a failure. Vivian longs to break free of the "oughtta's" that control her life, but she is just beginning to see how she might *choose* to respond differently. The more she understands about what is behind her easily triggered reactions, the more she senses that choosing to respond in a different manner is within her power. For the moment, though, she is still having trouble letting the past go and getting unstuck.

Vivian may be at the point in her journey where progress often seems to be two steps forward and one step backward. But she is beginning to look behind her emotions to see what past facts and realities they point to. She's beginning to give herself permission to re-evaluate those old messages and to make adjustments to make them relevant for today or to let them go and not be influenced by them any longer. She is beginning to see that if she rejects old *responses* to her older sister's comments that she is not rejecting that sister, or the positive feelings from her childhood, or the experiences that link her to the mother she barely remembers but longs to connect to.

How We Get Stuck in Old Patterns

After our survival requirements for air, water and food are met, our experiences with fear and love in their many guises become prime motivators of our behavior. And these motivators act on the most important part of our existence—our relationship with others.

One function of the prime motivators is to provide signals that enable us to avoid danger. Fear or hurt, for example, can stimulate us to stand to defend ourselves (fight) or to move to protect ourselves (flight). For some of us, these experiences can be so overwhelming that we freeze with inaction, even if it causes harm to us. Positive experiences that make us feel loved and secure can help us learn skills to cope. Positive experiences also provide supportive encouragement.

As infants and children these experiences take place in the context of families. We learn from the significant others in our lives, starting with the indelible influence of our mothers and going on to that of our fathers, siblings and other significant surrogates. Later, our peers play a role. All these significant others knowingly or unknowingly teach us about ourselves through our experiences with them.

As infants, attachment to our primary caregiver, usually Mom, is crucial to early development because this attachment or bonding shapes a perception of acceptance, love, and worth. These experiences provide the framework that enables us to become who we are. The more solid and positive the attachment, the better we're able to reach our fullest potential for the challenges of life. Anything short of that may be sufficient for life, but not really adequate for reaching our fullest potential.

Our attachment to mother (or dad or primary caregiver) grounds us in our own identity. As we connect or form attachment with "mom," we are learning attachment to ourselves. We are freed to *be*. If we don't experience a firm attachment early, we tend to search ceaselessly for a surrogate or substitute. The substitutes may take the form of over pursuit of work, adult hobbies or toys, chemical dependencies or lifestyle addictions, even religious zeal.

Our mothers, fathers, and families also teach us how to live with others, an ability psychologists call *socialization*. The nature of human reality is that we are social beings who are hard-wired to grow and function in social relationships—in community. The positive and negative experiences in the dynamic interplay of these relationships shape our sense of ourselves, our feelings, our view of others, and our modes of coping with whatever experience brings. In these relationships and their interactions, therefore, lie memories of the origins of many of our hurts.

As part of maturing, each individual realizes an inner need to be a separate person, to take control of one's identity, to set different boundaries to protect oneself against being vulnerable to others, and to establish one's independence. And this stage opens new opportunities for support or conflict with those we care about.

It's important to understand how and why our own unique methods of living life and pursuing life developed and why and how they are ultimately important to us. When we see ourselves in a clearer light, we are then better able to see our options for change and make clearer choices for change. We can then be free to drop the accumulating hurts, frustrations, and angers.

Our response to individual hurts or negative experiences alone doesn't inflict the injury. Instead multiple injuries produce a cumulative effect. As we accumulate negative hits over months and years, they function much like an inoculation or vaccination for pain. This pain inoculation brands the lesson into us, triggering a chronic, toxic reaction any time we encounter an actual negative experience or our brain's emotional memory center processes an experience as negative. It's important to understand at this point that, given the complexity of human psychology, the positive or loving intent of the other individuals involved in any given experience does not necessarily mean that we perceive it as they intend— or, indeed, as it actually is or was. I call these trigger points *buttons*.

Buttons and Boundaries

What actions or events push anyone's buttons? Although one person's buttons differ from another's, buttons are usually triggered when personal boundaries are violated. Boundaries, in this sense, refer to how we define ourselves in relation to others. Such boundaries are spatial—what we mean when we say "my space" vs. "your space" or "our space" vs. "their space." Such relational boundaries typically describe emotional, psychological, and intellectual space that often may be backed up by physical space.

Our view of our space in relation to the space of others determines how we view our separateness from others, which can be healthy or not. After all, is it OK for me to reach outside my space into another's? How do I receive the concept that my space does not extend beyond the limits of my own cylinder, so to speak? This concept includes how I view my space, your space, what is allowed as an extension of self, essentially what's mine and what's yours. Can we each be separate and yet play, live, or exist compatibly together? These are all part of the working model of relating to others that we develop starting during infancy.

There are also spaces bound within us that are important to understand and clarify conceptually. My arm, for instance, is an important part of me, but isn't *me*. And so, the discovery of a disease within me doesn't change who I am any more than my hammer-smashed, throbbing, red, painful thumb does. If I'm anxious, then it's okay to view myself as the same me who also happens to have developed anxiety that I need to attend to. As previously stated, I am not my heart attack. These distinctions are important, for as much as the disease is part of me, impossible to escape from and sort of in my face with pain, i.e., headache, neck pain, or cancer and occupying my mind with misery, I can maintain a healthy separateness from it and still be *me*. With this distinction, I can better relate to each health condition, face the challenge it presents, and keep my focus on the task before me or whatever else life presents.

Buttons related to the security and comfort of my space as well as to any threats to it are formed early in life. Our buttons approach the essence of our relationships. Buttons, like boundaries, are part of our personalities, a direct extension of our upbringing. Those buttons specifically tie together the fabrics of our training and experience over the whole course of our lives. As the buttons appear in our training, we unconsciously perceive them as strategically placed protective devices defending us against a hostile world. Some buttons help divert the reaction outward, some inward and others seem designed to sweep the reaction right into our defense systems. In the process of living and growing, boundaries are breached and buttons are activated, amplifying the events and further sensitizing us and honing our behavioral response to those types of experiences.

As we grow from infancy into childhood, working to establish ourselves as distinct, independent selves, we human beings are busy engaging others and the world in order to learn about ourselves. From observing others and from processing our own experiences we create working models for behavior. We learn how to act outwardly and inwardly. We refine resistance, anger and wall-building along with positive traits. As we practice behaving as we're labeled or rebelling against labels, as we test and retest boundaries, as we incorporate into our working model the many messages we hear (some from others and many self-messages from processing experience), we set up our many buttons. Through the years, we continue to refine the ways we relate to others while basically retaining the original working model, with both its positive and negative baggage.

Bluffing Your Way through Life and Accepting Labels

Another stumbling block that relates to our feelings and the messages that we've received about ourselves is feeling like we somehow do not deserve our success or achievement or that we are "living a lie." One aspect of this is often called the *imposter syndrome* because we feel inadequate or that we haven't actually earned the positive outcomes (doing well in school or business, being well liked, being judged intelligent or able by those with whom we work). Many of these feelings are related to labels—expectations that others have set for us, that we perceive that others have set for us, or that emerge from self-messages.

A label is usually short-hand for a particular image of one's self. For example, a parent may say something like "that's my Big Boy or Big Girl" when a small child achieves an expectation such as not crying after a fall. The process of growing up and maturing is loaded with opportunities for labeling. Parents, siblings, playmates, teachers and others with whom we interact are constantly articulating images of who we are—these images can work positively or negatively depending on where we are emotionally and how we are helped to handle them.

For instance, academically bright parents often unconsciously expect that their child will be intelligent and high achieving rather than seeing the child as a separate person whose unique talents and interests need to be explored and affirmed and whose own feelings, desires, and fears need to be respected in the nurturing, mentoring and disciplining process.

A label can also give us a way out of choosing to change when we feel insecure. Typically, a label that characterizes a situation or condition pins it down and brings satisfaction. It anchors us in time, and gives us an excuse for not moving forward or even for going backward, thus stunting our growth.

Sid's Story

Sid, a 50-year-old participant in a support group for men recovering from heart events, is a good case in point. By his own description, Sid grew up thinking he was royalty. His parents made sure that he had everything he needed to excel in school, social life, and work. His dad, in particular, was always available and ready with advice, instruction and supervision for schoolwork and scouting and other activities during his childhood and teen years. His parents saw that he had golf lessons and tennis lessons—something most of his peers couldn't afford. When it came time for college, Sid's dad chose the school and advised him to study business—a useful major when he entered the family business.

CHOICES

And, just as expected, Sid entered the business, where his dad told him exactly what to do and when to do it, never asking Sid what he thought about business or anything else. Sid's dad once explained that his intent was to save Sid from having to experience the hardships he had gone through, to relieve him of that burden. Because Sid was completely accustomed to asking his dad's advice in everything and following instructions and being praised for doing so, this course of affairs seemed normal. Just as normal as having his mother, and later his wife, take care of all his home and personal needs.

Then after Sid had been in the family business for about seven years, his father died unexpectedly. Suddenly, Sid literally had to take care of business by himself. He felt deserted. Without any training or experience in making business decisions, he struggled. The stress was tremendous. He felt inadequate and ill-equipped and undeserving; he was sure he'd be a disappointment to his father. But he knew his dad would want him to carry on the business, so he did. In fact, he did it well—and the business actually grew.

But secretly, Sid kept expecting things to go wrong. Drinking helped lessen the stress. Drinking a little more helped him sleep at night. Drinking helped keep him from acknowledging a slow anger at how much his dad had controlled him, never asked for or encouraged him to think independently, and in a sense had rejected him and set him up for a fall. Because Sid drank too much, ate poorly (lots of fatty comfort food), and shunned physical activity, he soon acquired a whole host of risk factors—overweight, high blood pressure, high cholesterol—that are associated with heart disease and diabetes.

After a fairly mild heart attack, Sid became furious with the rehab team who were encouraging him to follow a more prudent lifestyle. "I'm not going to change anything," he shouted; "I like my life. I like things the way they are. I'm not changing!" With some help in support group, however, Sid discovered that underneath his adamant desire not to change was the fear that he couldn't do it successfully.

Sid's biggest enemy was the labels that he had accepted as his self-concept. And what were these labels? That he was unable to perform. That he couldn't do new tasks without someone watching over his shoulder and advising. That he could not think through difficult concepts or logically solve problems on his own. That he was a phony, an imposter, who masqueraded as independent when he really felt dependent on others for everything. Slowly Sid realized that he was caught in the trap of his father's image of him, not his own. Slowly, he realized that his deepest desire was to be himself.

As a result of being forced by poor health to stop and examine his life, Sid discovered that personal history produces personal mindsets and maps for behavior that we tend not to examine. He also discovered that the true imposter is that aspect of self that avoids looking honestly at feelings to discover the facts behind them.

When Sid identified his skills and explored the real accomplishments of his life, he realized that although much had been negative in his working relationship with his dad, he had learned to pay attention, to absorb information and to put it to work in a disciplined way and those were his talents, his achievements alone. And they were a good foundation for choosing to be the independent person he wished to be. With this foundation he was able to stop drinking, to modify his lifestyle, and more important to build more rewarding relationships with his wife and children.

Through this process Sid discovered one of the key benefits of exploring feelings as guides to the facts behind them:

> *You can rise to your stars—your true or ideal identity,*
> *but you live down to your labels.*

Most important, Sid like Dave and Vivian discovered that you can *choose* to change.

What Choice Has to Do with It

Those who cannot remember the past are condemned to repeat it.
        —Santayana, 20th century American philosopher

When you understand the root causes of behavior, you have the power to choose new responses. In fact, we can summarize some of the important messages from our examples and discussion in a couple of simple diagrams.

You are what you
- think
- feel
- believe
- eat
- do

The typical discussion of the risk factors for heart disease, cancer, hypertension, diabetes and other chronic conditions focuses on what you eat and do. And popular media harp on the consequences of poor lifestyle choices—high fat diet, lack of exercise, for instance. But these health habits grow out of what we think, feel, and believe deep inside.

You are
- how you see yourself
- how you interpret your world
- what you don't like
- what you criticize in others
- what you dream of becoming

You can not know the accurate answers to these topics unless you face your feelings and use them as cues to lead you to the facts behind your choices and behaviors. Ignoring feelings or pushing them under the surface simply leads to continued problems.

In the next chapter, we will explore practical techniques that will help you go "back to the future" to free yourself for joyful and full living.

5

Dive, Dive, Dive

Practical Techniques for Identifying the Facts Behind the Feelings

In this chapter

Feelings can cue you to danger, stimulate you to move to safety, and enable you to change positively, but only if you "listen" below the surface. Only you can open yourself to the process and only you can find the facts.

This chapter shows you how to use specific techniques such as "Back to the Present" and "Story Telling" to dig safely, accurately, and productively into the facts behind your feelings. These are simple techniques that you can use over and over to dig down to the depths needed to go below your protective layers to uncover the "real you."

You use these techniques privately for yourself and at your own speed. Using these exercises within a planned program will help you breakthrough to new insights and choices.

"Ah, yes, I remember it well"

Do you remember that scene from the film musical *Gigi*, when Gigi's grandmother and the boulevardier played by Maurice Chevalier reminisce about their youthful romance, and each remembers the same events somewhat differently? "Ah, yes, I remember it well" goes the gently ironic tagline of their amusing duet.

Memory is a tricky thing. If you and I go to a movie or ballgame, then write down the highlights, the basic outline of events in our accounts may be similar, but our observations of what was important will differ. Because memory is so tricky, and so subjective, you may be concerned if you use feelings as cues to help identify the facts behind them that what you discover may be misleading. Let me assure you that all the ideas and techniques in this chapter recognize that memories are personal and subjective, not objective. But your personal perceptions and the feelings or emotions connected to them are in themselves *facts*.

The techniques in this chapter provide a structure to help you look behind personal perceptions and feelings. As you fold back the layers or pull together the intertwining pieces using memories and experiences, you'll look at what's happening inside, or has happened, from many different angles.

Memory is also tricky because events, experiences, or perceptions that may be important to why we feel and act as we do tend to hide—almost as if the memory centers of our brains store the "reports" sideways so that only the thin edges are visible. This is particularly true if the events remembered were negative. The techniques in this chapter can help you get beyond these barriers without giving up personal control. Remember that the primary goal of using feelings to find the facts is to free yourself to choose to become the person you want to be.

We can't live *by* our feelings, we can only learn to live *with* them, to learn to trust them as cues, and to use them as tools to guide us back to the facts (about ourselves and others). Learning to use your feelings in this way will help you accomplish several important goals:

- To make choices based upon facts, not emotions
- To keep doors to relationships open
- To evaluate emotions and personal history with distance to avoid making irrational decisions today based on what may have been rational choices in the past.

But achieving these goals is the focus of Chapter 9. Before you can use your feelings as cues to growth and change, you need to dive deep into your mind and memories to find out what's going on behind those feelings.

What Does It Take to Go There?

So how do we get into your head? *We* don't. Only *you* can. In the following pages, I will share several structured techniques that you can use, first, to take you below the surface (not always easy) and, second, to guide your exploration. Your objective is to look behind your current experiences and feelings to identify some of the roots or sources of your working model for relating to others as well as for your mindset, beliefs, and values.

Before you take the plunge, however, you need some "equipment" for diving into the formative experiences and memories behind your feelings.

Requirement 1: A softened heart.

I like this image because it represents an openness or willingness to explore and change. The fact that you are reading this book, even if you are skeptical, suggests that you are open to exploring new possibilities that may help you achieve the freedom you seek.

In addition, there are times in our lives that are usually accompanied with softened hearts—times when we are open to personal change. These times include such important mountain-top moments as falling in love, marriage, the birth of new child, or even starting a new job or career. These heart-softened times can also include experiences of loss or great crisis such as the death of a loved one, a health crisis (for instance, a heart attack, cancer diagnosis, or life-threatening illness or accident), or a job loss or change.

Requirement 2: Commitment of time

Most things worth doing take more than 30 seconds once a week. Even an occasional 30 minutes isn't enough. If you are serious about discovering the hidden messages that are trapping you into recycling negative, imprisoning behaviors, then you will need to set aside time to work regularly. Why not make an appointment with yourself? A new practice usually takes at least thirty days to become established routine. At first, you may require only ten or fifteen minutes a session. Then as you get into practice, you may wish to spend thirty to sixty minutes a session. In addition to "appointments" during your regular daily schedule, you could take advantage of other "down times" such as waits in airports for flights, time on flights, or "hotel-time" on business trips.

Requirement 3: Commitment to explore, not to judge

When anyone starts exploring feelings, the first temptation may be to look at what's wrong with others outside oneself. But don't go there. The purpose of these techniques is to look *within yourself* without standing in judgment—to find the facts about yourself and your perceptions, your relationships and experiences with others. Blame has no part in this "game." Understanding and growth are your goal.

Requirement 4: Patience—with yourself and others

None of us became our present selves or reached our current circumstances in a day. Not even in a few months or years. Major positive growth won't come instantaneously, either. Many positive things can happen quickly, but there will also be moments of frustration or times when it seems like you aren't getting anywhere. That's the time to remind yourself to cut yourself some slack, to have patience, and to stay with the program. It will work.

How To Use The Techniques—An Overview

I don't know about your personal history but mine is lengthy and full of events. If I thought I had to look at everything at once, I'd be overwhelmed. That's where the techniques and processes presented in this chapter come in. They provide a structure to focus and limit your exploration so that you get the most out of your work.

The techniques for looking behind your current feelings to find the facts begin with two general exercises designed to help you explore specific experiences and feelings. When you feel ready to start putting all the pieces together, you can use the process presented in the second section. To get an idea of how the techniques flow together I suggest that you read through the whole chapter first, then begin with either starting technique—"back to the present" or "storytelling"—whichever seems right for you at the time. At the end of chapter 9, I have also provided a calendar of possible working topics for many weeks, but before you go there, I suggest that you try the techniques as described in the next few pages.

Because anger is a major cloaking emotion that everyone experiences, you may wish to go ahead to read Chapter 6, which offers some exercises for exploring how you experience and re- spond to anger. In fact, it's okay to start with the exercises about anger and then use this chapter's techniques to deepen or expand your exploration. One of the nice things about the techniques and tools in these chapters, besides their simplicity, is that you can use them over and over. In fact, that's the only way to get any real benefit from them. Another nice thing is that you can adapt them to fit your personal style.

Getting Started—Finding and Defining Your Feelings

Both of the following exercises ask you to visualize a lot. Some people find it helpful to imagine they are creating or playing a videotape in their head. I recommend that you do these exercises in writing (paper or computerized journal). Writing your experiences, images and thoughts down allows you to preserve continuity and to go back to ideas from one session to another. It also frees you up to roam as far as your thoughts take you because you won't lose an idea or image if you've written it down. Writing it down makes the memory or experience concrete, frees it up, and allows you to put it outside yourself for easier examination. Writing your thoughts down also makes it easier to put them together in the second step. Writing in the first person ("I") is preferred. However, as you begin the process, it may be easier for you to begin writing your stories in the third person ("he" or "she"). Then, later you'll easily be able to switch to the more personal first person to complete the process.

CHOICES

Technique 1: Back to the Present

This simple exercise can be (and should be) used over and over. Once you've practiced the technique, you'll find that you can use it in any circumstance to examine your feelings to quickly identify "what's going on" —the motivating facts—behind your feelings and actions. You can download worksheets for this exercise from the book's website: www.choices-letstalk.com.

Set up

Find a comfortable environment, in safe harbor. It could be a favorite chair in a room by yourself, a snug seat at a favorite coffee shop, a quiet place outdoors, or any spot where you feel comfortable and secure and where you won't be interrupted. You might choose a straight-backed chair—comfort is fine, lounging is not.
Your approach is not whining, not having a pity-party, and not anxious. I suggest that you write in a journal (paper or computer) but you don't have to.

Do it

1. Relax and clear your mind. You may wish to close your eyes. Imagine a blank screen or sheet of paper, a clear sky, a warm gray expanse—anything that gently clears your mind. Now let the events and thoughts of your day drift in. You might think of this as running a videotape. Describe your day or an event or a situation during the day—whatever comes to mind first is fine.

2. Don't worry about trying to focus on your feelings —just tell what happened. In telling about the event(s), your feelings will appear at the appropriate time in the context of your story. You must wait on them. You might close your eyes and imagine an elevator gently lifting up some scene into your consciousness.

   When these emotions come, they will signal their presence. You might just have a sense of it, or you might feel a stirring of anger or pleasure or even a physical sensation such as clearing your throat, feeling flushed, choking up a little, or a faster heart beat. When you begin to describe an emotion or give an event a value, that's a signal to start diving deeper.

3. Even if you don't immediately identify a feeling with an event or situation. The fact that it stood out in your day suggests clearly that it has feelings attached to it. Select a stand-out event.

4. When you've identified this event, would you describe it as positive or negative? Why? What other events does it remind you of in the past? Go back as far as you can. Follow the thread into childhood events if possible, matching the current event with similar events in your past. These may be events with similar circumstances or simply similar "feels" to them.

5. Listen to the messages attached to the events. What are they? What issues do they raise? What values do these messages reflect? How do these embedded values relate to your personal values and beliefs today? How are the messages attached to the events, situations and persons? Is your feeling, action, or behavior being dictated by some other voice (whose?) or your own?

6. You may wish to use the four squares of the Johari's window to look at the experience from different points of view. What is clear to everybody? What do you see that is hidden from others? What might others see about you that has perhaps been hidden from you until you began to examine the experience more deeply? Do you discern any possible areas where facts might be deeply buried and hidden from both you and others?

7. By asking yourself questions like those above and reflecting without pressure on the events, your past will begin to teach you, give you understanding and provide you with data

about yourself. These are the facts you need to re-evaluate in order to determine how rational your past decisions and choices were.

8. You can then fast-forward those decisions and choices to your present and rethink them. Do they still reflect values and beliefs you'd like to keep or do you want to develop new or updated standards that are more appropriate for your experiences, goals, and growth today? Have you already developed some of these new or updated standards? Would you choose to free yourself from any message, belief or value? Which one(s)? Why? What belief or value would you choose instead? Write these goals down. Again using the four squares of the Johari's window may help you organize your reflections.

Technique 2: Storytelling

The exercise I call "storytelling" is another good way to dive below your defenses and identify past experiences with positive and negative messages that help shape your current feelings and behaviors.

Set up

Find a comfortable environment, where you can sit and write comfortably and where you won't be interrupted.

Your approach is not whining, not having a pity-party, and not anxious. This technique is most effective when you actually write in a journal (paper or computer).

Do it

The following paired phrases are springboards that are designed to help you dive back into past experiences or stories. You'll notice that each pair of phrases contains one negative prompt and one positive prompt—always do both.

When you read each phrase, what event or story from your past comes to mind? Don't judge or evaluate at this point, just let an idea, association, or picture float up. Note that idea, event or image down and describe it. Then go to the other phrase and repeat the process. After you've described the events, use the set of questions below to identify the feelings and the facts that are revealed in these Stories. Downloadable worksheets are on www.choices-letstalk.com.

You can start with any pair of phrases that strikes you.

1. My biggest fight/conflict with a parent
    A special moment with a parent.

2. My biggest fight/conflict with a sibling (or friend)
    A special moment with a sibling (or friend)

3. A scary moment in childhood
    A comforting, secure moment in childhood

4. Losing
    Winning

5. A time of loneliness
    A time of friendship/belonging

6. The worst present/birthday I ever had
    The best present/birthday I ever had

7. A time I was punished unfairly
    A time I was rewarded

8. A time I was misunderstood
    A time I was appreciated

9. A moment of family togetherness
    A moment of family struggle or disruption

10. A family celebration
    A family fight

11. Holiday memories to cherish
    Holiday memories to forget

12. Grief
    Joy

13. Sweet revenge
    A mouthful of ashes

14. A moment of rejection
    A moment of praise

15. A grudge I can't let go
    A moment of giving that made me feel good

16. An experience I feel proud of
    An experience I'm ashamed of

When you've described the events, listen to the messages attached to the events.

- What are they?
- What issues do they raise?
- What values do these messages reflect?
- How do these embedded values relate to your personal values and beliefs today?
- How are the messages attached to the events, situations and persons?
- Is your feeling, action, or behavior being dictated by some other voice (whose?) or your own?

You may wish to use the four squares of Johari's window to look at the experience from different points of view. What is clear to everybody? What do you see that is hidden from others? What might others see about you that has perhaps been hidden from you till you began to examine the experience more deeply? Do you discern any possible areas where facts might be deeply buried and hidden from both you and others?

By asking yourself questions like those above and reflecting without pressure on the events, your past will begin to teach you, give you understanding, and provide you with data about yourself. These are the facts you need to re-evaluate to determine how rational your past decisions and choices were.

You can then fast-forward those decisions and choices to your present and rethink them.

- Do they still reflect values and beliefs you'd like to keep or do you want to develop new or updated standards that are more appropriate for your experiences, goals, and growth today?
- Have you already developed some of these new or updated standards?
- Would you choose to free yourself from any message, belief or value?
- Which one(s)? Why?
- What belief or value would you choose instead? Write these goals down.

Putting It All Together

Using the other exercises in this chapter prepares you for "Putting It All Together." In the earlier exercises you've been looking at particular events to discover the facts behind those memories and associated feelings. In this larger exercise, you will use the same techniques of story telling to begin to draw all the threads together and look at your total story. You will also use the specific events you've identified earlier as building blocks for this exercise. Your end objective is to clarify the whole picture of where you've been, what messages and values have kept you stuck, and where you want to go and grow.

There are three steps:
1. Think it through, write it down, discuss it (even if just with yourself)
2. Dissect it
3. Grade it (without blame)

Step 1: Think it through, write it down, discuss it

Dreams don't come true by themselves. Most of us may have dreamed a lot about life with little experience in essential planning or in thinking how to make the dreams reality. Planning and implementation start with memory and analysis.

The process is simple: Write your whole story down (in concrete form). Insert stories from your previous exercises as they show up in the timeline of your life. You can tell your story from beginning to end—or you can jump around in time—concentrating on your most vivid memories and then branching out from there. Or you might focus on one type of story at a time, such as "experiences that make me mad" or "events that make me feel connected." In other words, you can start with what's bothering you most right now.

As you think of details, remember that our lives are about people and our relationships with them. After you get your story on paper (or in the computer), read it straight through. Then reread it, asking yourself if your narrative represents actual events and experiences as clearly and accurately as possible. Edit and add until it does.

As you review your story, pinpoint the anger in your experiences, because those episodes may be the key to the door to your deeper and more accurate memories.

As you go along, also list any messages, buttons, and labels that pop up. Thinking more deeply about these can unearth other experiences and voices from your past. Add these new events to your story.

At first, the task of writing down your whole life can seem daunting. It's natural to think, "I don't want to go there. The task is too big. I'm also scared of what might turn up." Like one person I know, you might even use a weather metaphor: 'Let's not go there; the weather's too bad."

Well, I'm glad you brought up the weather. The Scandinavians have a very practical approach to extreme cold or terrible weather. There's no such thing as bad weather, they say, only bad choices of clothing!

What a useful concept that is for this exercise. In your life you probably have selected pieces of the right clothing as well as plenty of inadequate clothing to help handle the storms and heatwaves of life as well as the ordinary nothing-much-is-happening kind of daily weather.

As you look at your story, what clothing—values and beliefs—have you chosen wisely? Which would you change? What "messages" and "labels" have you put on that don't really fit? Why? What new messages or values or qualities would you choose? Have you already chosen some of these?

The messages, labels and unrealistic expectations distance us from the present moment and bind us to the "me" mode, maintaining our self-centeredness, calling up our pride and stubbornness. Messages and labels make us resist change and growth. In fact, unless you have evaluated those messages and labels and made new choices, those people who taught you the outworn messages and labels still rule you (sometimes even from the grave).

How can you tell if those old messages are still exerting their control? How about if you find yourself saying, "It's too much trouble," "it's too hard for me," "I don't have the energy," "I don't have time," or "I can't carry all that load alone"? Freedom enables us to shed these blocks.

Step 2: Dissect it

In order to see more clearly what's really going on in your stories—the facts behind the feelings—you need to be able to distance yourself from them a little. That's not easy. But writing them down is the first step. The next step is to mentally remove yourself from the center of the drama and begin to look at it from the outside. Break down the story into the players and the elements in the event. Remember you're looking for the facts, not trying to place blame on anyone.

Suggested stories to dissect

As you look over your whole history, you may find that two types of stories offer the most effective places to begin:

- Very vivid events in which you have a central role. Other ways to describe such vivid events include "that story... is still fresh, ...still takes my breath away, ...still makes me angry (or sad, or choked up) every time I think about it, or ...seems like yesterday"

- An event from a family tradition or holiday. Such times are notoriously stressful partly because gathering family and friends together includes the dynamics of many relationships. And remember relationships are at the heart of the work you're trying to do.

Questions to guide your dissection

For each event you select, describe the following:
- Who are the participants in the event (include yourself)? How is each participant related to you (sibling, parent, aunt, cousin, family friend, etc.)?
- What lesson was being taught or what were you learning in this event?
- What way was that lesson being taught?
- What events or facts (such as ongoing circumstances in the family) were behind it?
- What "voices" are you hearing in the event?
- What response did you make to the "lesson"?
- How did/do you feel about that?
- As best as you can, describe the scene from the perspective of each of the other participants—a parent, teacher, brother, sister, friend, etc.
- What are the lessons from their point of view, in your opinion?
- Are you still using any of these lessons to shape/determine your behavior? Do you feel they are still appropriate or not? Why or why not?

As you did in earlier exercises, it may be useful to use the Johari's window to help you look at the experiences from different points of view.

Step 3: Grade it

Review your stories and grade them by the quality and quantity of positive references (versus negative). Give primary attention to your interactions and relationships with the other participants in each story.

Look at a specific story (or even several related stories): How do you score the way you were treated by each person influencing your upbringing? Use a scale of 1 to 10 where 10 is "perfectly positive" and 1 is "perfectly terrible."

Try to answer these questions for each individual in each event:
- Were they kind?
- Did they speak softly and calmly or were they short, irritated, or angry?
- Did they encourage you as you grew in various tasks?
- Did they listen to you and hear you?
- Did they voice or show approval of you?
- Did they set clear boundaries? Did they clarify those boundaries in positive ways?
- Were they consistent with their treatment of you and did you look forward to spending time with them? Was that time together fun or otherwise meaningful?

Using your answers and scores decide what they indicate about what was positive and negative in the interaction. By analyzing what's going on and "grading" the positive quality of several events, you can more accurately understand how you were treated in your upbringing. You can observe the difference between warmth and coolness, the influence of anger, the place for sternness and boundary setting, the difference between discipline and punishment (without anger) given by those who parented you.

You also need to ask what other variables are at work in any event that could make the picture more complex. Look at the dynamics between other individuals in the event. Also put the events in the context of then and now.
- What was the bigger picture then?
- What is the bigger picture for you now?
- How do all the events flow together?
- What has changed?
- Do you feel that the "message teachers" gave you permission to take their "rules" or "philosophies" forward as you grew?
- Did the messages affirm or ignore your right and need to re-evaluate and decide to keep or change aspects of the working models you learned? What are your options now?

CHOICES

As you look at the bigger picture, acknowledge that you have the freedom to choose and that choosing differently is not rejecting those you care about. Begin to think about areas where you'd like to make new choices and areas where you'd like to affirm positive models from the past.

What to Do with What You Learn with These Techniques

Where will you be when you finish this chapter? And what are the next steps? If you have been serious about your work and given enough scope to your work, you should begin to see certain patterns emerging that help you put into words the reasons why you act as you do and why those behaviors, so often recycled and worn-out, aren't working any more. You'll see the probable origins of many variables that have made up your working model for living. These variables include your perceptions, coping skills, adaptability, values, thoughts, beliefs, and actions. All these perceptions provide the facts that you can use to help you be your true self and nurture the relationships you want to have. Later in the book, Chapter 9 shows you how to put your facts to work for yourself today.

But before you go to Chapter 9, I'd urge you to go straight on to Chapter 6 on anger. After engaging seriously in an exploration of anger, most people find that anger (often buried anger or redirected anger) is playing a bigger role in their responses and reactions to stress and life than they thought.

After you've worked through Chapters 6 and 9, I've provided a 36-week long calendar of possible topics that you can use as a framework for exploring all that you need to learn and for making choices for change and growth.

Before we move on, one more thought may help you going forward. Your feelings as cues are more accurate the instant they appear, so increase your awareness of them and listen-up to what they're telling you. This earliest assessment before the brain mechanisms build the full perceptual picture is what you're to pay attention to. These are the moments the cue is friend, that is, it's a window through which to peer into your true reaction, the feelings that respond before the baggage is added and the message becomes tainted, less objective and less accurate.

6

Climbing Off the Anger Ladder

In this chapter

What is anger? What are its roots?

Practical techniques for identifying what's behind the anger in your life

How to choose alternative, positive coping strategies

In previous chapters, I've talked about anger as one of the powerful feelings that can help lead us to the facts about our experiences and behaviors. I've also described anger as a "cloaking" or "secondary" emotion that hides another emotion such as fear or hurt. It's also true that anger itself is often a hidden emotion. Although most of us know when we are experiencing rage or are "shouting mad," we may not recognize some of the other guises of anger, particularly the anger that expresses itself as depression, cynicism or sarcastic joking, or even boredom. In this chapter, I want us to look together more closely at anger, the ways it may play a role in your life and negatively affect your relationships. Then we'll turn to how you can climb off the anger ladder and choose more effective ways of responding to situations and actions that currently anger you.

Defining Anger and the Anger Ladder

Just what is anger? Like some other important things in life, anger may be something that you feel you have a hard time defining in words but you know what it is when you see it. Everyone recognizes *rage* as anger. But just how many other forms can you think of? To help, here's a list of behaviors that can express anger. The list is presented as a ladder with the most negative anger responses placed toward the top and the most positive or constructive responses placed at the bottom. Be aware, too, that the list is representative rather than all inclusive of anger responses.

ANGER LADDER

Negative Response ↑

Physical abuse
Emotionally destructive behavior
Verbal abuse
Destroying property
Throwing objects
Expressing unrelated complaints
Displacing anger onto other
Cursing
Unpleasant and loud behavior
Passive-aggressive behavior
Thinking logically and constructively
Holding to the primary complaint
Focusing anger on source only
Seeking resolution
Seeking resolution in a respectful manner

Positive response ↓

It's not hard to spot the anger or rage behind most of the negative behaviors on this anger ladder. But what are some of the many other types or manifestations of feelings that at their essence are anger? Take a look at some of these terms associated with anger (that produce behaviors somewhere on the anger ladder).

- agitated
- irritated
- annoyed

- disgusted
- critical
- frustrated
- fed up
- ticked off
- put out
- resentful
- impatient
- seething
- uptight
- worked-up
- perturbed
- aggressive
- hot under the collar
- critical
- envious
- bitter
- sarcastic
- hostile
- bored
- riled
- sore
- livid
- furious
- mad
- outraged
- irate

These varying descriptive terms indicate not only the level of anger we may be experiencing but also the varying levels of control we may have over the anger response. In some of these expressions, anger may also be more hidden than open, such as when anger expresses itself in bitterness or boredom or in sarcastic joking.

As children we usually learn that angry feelings are undesirable, perhaps even "bad" feelings—certainly they are something we are taught that we should avoid having (an impossible task) or if we do have them, we should not express them. All too often, however, rather than learning to control anger by understanding it and resolving the causes or understanding them and letting go, we learn to repress our awareness of our angry feelings.

Then, as Freud once observed, anger is like the smoke in an old-fashioned wood stove, if the smoke (anger) can't go up the chimney (the proper release) then it leaks out of the stove in unintended ways with negative consequences such as smoking up the room where people are trying to breathe. Here are just a few of the behaviors that may signal hidden anger, among other feelings.

- liking sadistic or ironic humor
- sarcasm, cynicism or flippancy in conversation
- grumpiness
- defensiveness
- perpetual or habitual lateness
- overpoliteness, constant cheerfulness and attitude of "grin and bear it"
- frequent sighing
- boredom, apathy, loss of interest in things you are usually enthusiastic about
- procrastination in the completion of imposed tasks
- smiling while hurting
- excessive irritability over trifles
- excessive sleeping; clenching or grinding teeth, especially while sleeping
- feeling down for extended periods for no reason (depression)
- waking up tired rather than refreshed
- chronically stiff or sore neck or shoulder muscles (tension)

Anger Used as a Way of Life

We've each climbed the anger ladder many times. Used as a motivator, anger has been useful to everyone. It's one of the basic human emotions, for which we early learn various modes of expression and use. Anger, however, that persists unresolved and is used as a continuous defense can "bite the biter." Such anger is, in fact, toxic to the person it inhabits. It is a learned and reinforced defense. We've all witnessed temper tantrums that got children what they were demanding—and we thought how spoiled they were. Yet, too often we continue to use anger, perhaps adapting it or masking it, to get our way right up through adulthood. Using anger to get one's way, living on the top of the anger latter, often works—anger lets us influence and control others because they try to avoid it or appease it.

Too often, however, anger attracts more anger, usually of equal or escalating intensity—it doesn't just go away. It's usually absorbed, not blown off as much as we hope. Instead, it wells-up inside and erupts in its various guises from the "automated" mode that we've forged starting in childhood. Anger erupts more frequently when it's been fueled, fed, watered and fertilized by ongoing experiences. There's always, for example, someone around you can manipulate. You flip the bait, they react to it, and then the head-butting takes off. Such anger generates fear in the targeted person and produces stress for both the producer and the recipient.

From Anger to Angst

Anger as a way of life leads to what I call an "angst-prone life." Angst-prone persons excessively and indiscriminately practice grumpiness, sarcasm, cynicism, manipulation of others (rejecting others, shifting the blame, expressing disappointment or downgrading others), or spewing their moodiness, fussiness and free-flowing anger. The anger may not actually be aimed at others, but the angry angst-prone individual is insensitive to how their anger affects others. In turn, others (who often aren't aware of the bigger picture) receive the anger and angst, react to it, and perpetuate the process by stirring the angst pot.

Anger grows into a status of being angst-prone when it has an anxiety component (the dictionary definition of *angst*, in fact). Problems caused by anger and angst escalate when we have a sense that we are no longer in control, are threatened with losing control, or are playing catch-up to maintain control. Striving and struggling to maintain iron-grip control over everything takes an inordinate amount of energy—far above the normal amount required to live our lives. The more we struggle, the less we feel in control, the more angry and anxious we get, with the result that we may explode in various ways, grow depressed and anxious, or try to avoid stuff.

Often we try to bring our anger and angst under control simply by avoiding confrontation. But such avoidance can actually be a form of "stuffing" the negative emotion. Such stuffed anger often evolves into depression. If we don't resolve the issues that are causing the angst, if we're not really okay, then eventually we become resentful. Anger, though it may be hidden, then starts to drive our actions. Often we try to push away. Literally. We may drive like a banshee down the expressway, snipe verbally at family and coworkers, or seek comfort through unhealthy habits—actions which trigger the bodily responses that eventually generate hypertension, atrial fibrillation, aggravate heart disease, precipitate heart attacks and strokes—and on and on.

Anger as a way of life is a competitive and learned show of force that aims to affect others. It's commonly accompanied by control issues, demand for credit and recognition, lack of flexibility, difficulty with attachments, disinterest in change and a preference for age-old, original family-learned comforts of life rather than the opposites.

Why So Defensive? Why Defend Your Defensiveness?

What a grump! Surely, you're supporting a big, long-term investment that's fueling the energy necessary to sustain your attitudes and actions. And, all the negative energy is eating at you, you feel bad and have unresolved issues. You're caught in a vicious cycle. There's no way to find satisfaction, and your grumpiness is reinforcing the behavior. If you could only hurt the other equal to your hurt. But even then, it wouldn't satisfy, because the consequences to you both wouldn't justify any satisfaction.

Explore your feelings beneath your anger, for that's the source of your resistance representing your hurt. Once you identify that hurt and grief, then you can stop the chaos fueling the negative cycle. Only then could you begin the process that would allow you to see how many times you risked reaching out, and because of your ineffective techniques to which you've been blind, you failed to make amends. Your reach was blocked by the others' resistance to attacks encountered; as a result, your heart was impaled and you were wounded all the more. In these circumstances, one needs to be prepared and rehearsed to withstand the heat, for success is on the other side. Your task is to acknowledge and accept yourself, where you are, where you've been and to explore more for if you stay as you are, your decision-making and health are at risk.

What Can You Do to Climb off the Anger Ladder?

What can you do to stop the automated responses that lead to the angst-prone life?

First, you must define your anger. And look at where it feeds your angst. Otherwise, anger swirls in your mind and leaves you in chaos—something to be avoided. It's best to think it through—to get beneath it and discover the root causes of the pain, then address that. We have to turn anger and angst into something more tangible to get them out of our systems and out of our lives. It's something you can do only by choice. You have to face matters head-on to expose the anger and then uncover the underlying feelings to enable you to reach the hurt that drives the engine, generating the fear and anxiety.

Angst-proneness, by definition, is a mindset, or lens, that filters your view of other people and situations. Your own individual mindsets and filters grow out of your past experiences (those automated responses first learned in childhood) and your belief and value systems. So by analyzing and understanding what's going on under your anger and angst, you can make new choices. You can turn around 180 degrees and live in a totally new way. It won't be easy and it won't happen overnight, but you'll be surprised at how quickly you can begin to reap benefits.

So for peace of mind, better relationships and health, look around from your perch on the anger ladder, observe how lonely it really is up there and uncover the binding, blocking behaviors so that you can start climbing off the ladder. As you search for your feelings beneath the defenses and then dive deeper to understand yourself, you'll be better able to face yourself, the issues that underlie your health and disease and "fess up" to the need for change. Then you can dismantle the blocking behaviors that serve as obstacles to being your true self. These behaviors serve as defenses. They serve as armor placed between the people who hurt you and your vulnerable self, and they meld with your hurts and fears. Usually, they have become over the years automated behaviors—they protected you once, but have outworn their usefulness.

CHOICES

First Steps in Climbing off the Anger Ladder

Following three basic steps can help you begin to look at the role anger plays in your life and to define ways to climb down your own particular anger ladder.

1. First, recognize just what ways anger plays a role in your life. The exercises in Chapter 5 can help you explore this.
2. Next, own up to those feelings of anger—acknowledge "Yes, I do get angry. Nobody's doing it to me without my permission."
3. Finally, choose ways to respond to or act on the anger to discharge it or put it to work in a positive response to re-solve the situations or behaviors that provoked the anger.

You may find that the following worksheet "How do I respond to anger?" can help you begin to identify your feelings and some paths by which you can start to look for the facts behind these feelings.

HOW DO I RESPOND TO ANGER? A Worksheet

What makes me angry is . .

When I'm angry at someone, I usually . . .

After expressing my anger, I feel . . .

When others express anger towards me, I feel . . .

When I feel that way, I usually . . .

One thing that has made me angry this week was . . .

The way I handled that anger was to . . .

After expressing that anger, I felt . . .

If I could have responded differently, I would have . . .

After you have worked through these questions, you will have identified experiences from your daily life or past that you can begin to use in the exercises presented in chapters 5 and 9. Download a worksheet at www.choices-letstalk.com.

A Tip for Dealing with Anger in the Heat of the Moment

Such exercises are fine for the long-run, you say, but what do I do right now when anger begins to seethe up? If you feel that you need a tool to better handle your overt anger right now, then here are two techniques that may help you immediately:

1. Give yourself a "time out"

2. Use an *"I" statement* to explain what you are feeling to the other person(s).

Here's an example of how these techniques might work. Let's say that your spouse has failed to carry out a family task that you thought you'd both signed off on. You begin to boil because the failure is going to inconvenience the whole family, and, by damn, the same sort of thing happened in your parents' family and in your family it happened last week and several times before that. Time to tell yourself: Whoa…, chill. Take a deep breath, let it out, and withdraw. If you need to voice your problem, if it's not appropriate just to let it go for now, then make an "I" statement.

    For example, you might say, "I'm having a real problem with the fact that this _____ has not been done yet. I'd like to talk about how we can now get the thing done the best way, but not till I've cooled down." That's an *I statement* that makes a clear indication of how you are feeling but does not blame or name call. Saying something like, "Spouse, your failure to carry this agreed-on task out is really making me angry" is certainly clear about your feelings but it's a "you statement"—blame is placed. As such, it tends to fuel the angst not defuse it.

    Your *I statement* alone may open up unheated discussion, or certainly pave the way for a calm discussion when you've cooled down. During your "time out" work on letting the anger go, not on stuffing it.

CHOICES

The Benefits to Climbing Off the Anger Ladder

By staying off the anger ladder you avoid simply covering over the chronic wounds. Off the ladder and on solid ground, you can choose to open your wounds to the air, clean them, and allow them to heal. You do this by learning what's beneath your anger—your underlying feelings. It's possible that you're the only one who is aware of your tender sensitivities and the many hurts you've endured that fuel the habitual anger. You, therefore, won't change until you discover what roots (and branches) got you into trouble and what uprooting and pruning must be done for health to return. Though reluctant for change, most people will begin the process if they understand the negative side of no change. You also need to think about the positive side of change. Here's just one story about the difference even ONE SMALL change can make.

One small step off the anger ladder = one big gain in life: a true story

A business executive I'll call "Katherine" had toiled for years for one company. She knew her worth—her department consistently had higher production numbers than others, she was often first to volunteer for an extra assignment, and customer satisfaction with her unit was always high.

But neither her boss nor the company as a whole seemed to really value her contribution. Sure they dished out praise verbally, but her paycheck didn't confirm that high opinion, she felt. Although company performance had been good over the years, her raises had been sporadic and there'd been none lately. Because the company had grown from a small to a large firm rather haphazardly and control remained in the founding partners' hands, there was no official company policy or procedure related to compensation issues.

At some point Katherine decided that if she was ever going to get a raise, she'd have to ask for it. By this time she was fairly steamed at her boss and the general take-them-for-granted attitude of top management to employees. Sure, her department was happy and productive, but she did the stroking and looked after them. Nobody had gone to bat for her, however.

After much thought she decided to ask for a raise. She then did her homework preparing for the meeting. She anticipated that confronting her boss would be a challenge. So she honed her arguments and rehearsed her presentation more than a few times. Two days before her appointment, she shared her goal and strategy with a friend.

The friend listened carefully before responding. "I think you've really got your act together and all the facts, but you sound like you think your boss is a mean, old grump—an enemy even. I'm afraid that your attitude will seep through your presentation as an undercurrent of hostility. That might really hurt your case. What if you visualize your boss as receptive and understanding rather than assuming before you go in that he's a rock in the road that you'll have to shove out of the way?"

Katherine thought about what her friend had said. What harm would it do? Certainly, her boss fussed and fumed when she pushed him for support for projects or other employees, but with a good case he usually said yes. She resolved to see her boss as receptive, then practiced her presentation again with that in mind. What did she have to lose? (If that approach failed, she could always drop back and punt—with him as the football!)

The meeting occurred. Katherine presented her case to her boss, couching her arguments in collegial terms that anticipated his understanding. To her amazement, he matched her new mindset of him; he seemed to hear what she had to say. Even when he challenged the amount of her salary request, she presented her rebuttal in a positive manner without becoming upset and defensive. Even before his final answer, she had the fleeting thought of liking him. She was even more delighted when he agreed with her assessment and granted her raise; without her request, he even elevated her title to reflect the real responsibility she held in the company.

Looking back, she felt like she'd even enjoyed the experience. Being a swift learner, she started analyzing her negative and angry feelings when they occurred in other situations and relationships and experimented with using different mindsets.

CHOICES

Five years later after she'd first asked for the big raise, a young lady approached Katherine at a charity event and expressed the highest praise and gratitude for the influence she had had on her. Who was this young woman? Katherine hadn't a clue. A little tactful questioning elicited the reason. The younger woman had been present during that first big raise-request encounter. As the boss's secretary, she'd been present to take minutes of the session. Focused on her main mission, Katherine hadn't remembered her. But the young woman had been all eyes and ears. That one encounter provided the secretary with a new model and reset the standard for dealing with a potentially difficult exchange. Given the no-personnel-policy culture of the company, the secretary had eventually used Katherine's technique to ask for her own raise. Success again.

Success can be yours too. Understand what's going on and choose a new mindset. Climb down off the anger ladder and replace the "burn" with understanding and the ability to let go and go forward.

7

Wising Up without Wimping Out—Issues for Men

In this chapter

Growing up male in America all too often reinforces various attitudes that produce behaviors with negative consequences for health and relationships:

- I am my work

- Be a tough guy who embraces pain for gain

- Always keep a stiff upper lip. Never let'em see you sweat (or cry).

- I'm the king of my castle.

- Cut me a little slack. I work hard; I deserve it. Being a little wild is just being a man.

- Just do it the way I say.

Men have the opportunity to meld the wildness encouraged in boys with unexplored or unrealized tenderness to free themselves from the burdens of bravado and false ideas of leadership. Many men learn balance too late—after illness or misfortune strike—if they learn it at all. Men in America have heavy baggage to carry unless they choose to let it go.

This chapter guides men readers step-by-step through options for exploration and change. The greatest benefit: men can discover how much more in control they can be and how much better they can lead, if they learn to let go certain things and focus on being in the moment.

CHOICES
A Historical Perspective to Start

From the Bible, God made his covenant with Abraham, a man.

From the cradle of democracy, Aristotle asserted that man's seed produced the gift of life and woman's body served as only the vessel.

From antiquity, Rites of Passage originated to define boys' transformation into manhood. More accurately, the Rites served to shield and lift boys from tremendous anxiety experienced over separation from the stable and dependable life with their mothers.

From the earliest days of Western culture, manhood has been defined by other men, by what they do and the company they keep—it's a man's world.

> If John's wife had been sitting any closer he might have hit her. "That is *not* relevant!" he snapped at her, showing his teeth, with fire in his eyes. The incident lasted only a few seconds. But it was so vehement that I tensed, ready to intervene. His wife, however, didn't even flinch; she seemed to take his behavior as normal.
>
> John and his wife of forty-three years were in my office for the first visit after a referral to have John's heart problems evaluated. His burst of raw anger really startled me and made me fear for him.
>
> Four to six weeks later, after his work-up had been completed and we had clear direction for his treatment, John returned for a follow-up visit. He was alone this time and more relaxed. I brought up the incident with him. He said that he knew his wife was his friend and that the information she had given was helpful and important for his history and he was fortunate she was used to him, letting him get away with such behavior. Because their way of interacting was working for him, it was "Okay" he felt. John clearly had a clue about his behavior, knew he gets away with it, and rather enjoyed it, even flaunted it.

Guys are we caught in a curse? Or is it mostly the way we are brought up in our culture? Do we begin most conversations with our spouses or partners asserting our will or interests and explaining/defending our actions? Do we have to rule over all—especially our most loved ones, our spouses and children?

Think about it: Is life all about us? About being in charge? About winning? About being aggressive in seeking and getting what we want? Do we think that to be otherwise is to be less manly, less brave, less successful? Is this stance truly what we want life to be? Or are we trapped in an essentially false and destructive way of living? Have we thought enough about what's going on in our lives to know that we live in this way actually by *choice*?

Growing Up Male in America

What are you going to be when you grow up? As we guys grow, that looming question lies heavy on our minds. We are subtly and frequently reminded of it as we develop from boys to young men. Whatever our behavior as children, acting out wildly or not wildly enough, most of us boys are encouraged to avoid emotions and to suppress a more tender side. For example, calling certain activities or feelings "girlish" or "sissy" is one typical way that boys are channeled toward being "tough," supposedly to prepare us for an uncertain and threatening world in which we have to "succeed." But by such "toughening" and by cutting us slack for "boyish" behavior, our mentoring adults distract us from developing our feelings, from becoming as comfortable with our tender side as with our toughness or anger. This *training* prevents us from being able to express ourselves through effective communication.

In these ways, we learn to build armor to protect our hearts from threatening experiences in the world, and at the same time we learn to demand attention from others. These lessons learned in life's early experiences meld with socially accepted methods of expression to appear as competitiveness. Competition early in life produces both good and bad stress. The bad stress can become seeds of compulsions to action and competition when we become adults. However, competition has double edges, one side keeps one sharp, the other cuts sharply. What's cut is often our health.

By the time we men are well established in adulthood and have families of our own and careers to grow or maintain, we often find ourselves stuck in patterns that hurt rather than enhance our well-being.

CHOICES
Typical Ways Men Get Stuck

Here I offer you several thumbnail descriptions of some attitudes or points of view typical of men. These attitudes tend to produce stressful behavior that has negative consequences for your health and relationships.

- **I am my work.** "What are you going to be when you grow up?" As I just noted, guys live with this stressful question from the time that we are boys. Over the years, the question grows in significance —particularly if we don't have a ready answer or truthfully don't know. At some point the idea takes root that what we do—our work—is the most important thing about us. Gradually we learn to vest our identity in our work at the expense of seeing ourselves as whole apart from that job or career or profession.

- **Be a tough guy who endures pain for gain.** This attitude is all about winning—about success in achieving end goals. Gaining the goal is everything. It says men should take risks, stay tough, "play through pain" to gain the objective. Adopting this attitude of toughness is often a way of burying the fear that to do otherwise is to be a wimp. I see this attitude in patients who go at their cardiac rehab programs with a gung-ho intensity as if they need to prove that having had a heart attack has not made them somehow less a man. Such blind intensity in rehab or in work can create stress that undercuts achieving the goal.

- **Always keep a stiff upper lip. Never let'em see you sweat (or cry).** This attitude stuffs down feelings rather than expressing them appropriately or letting them go. It's closely related to enduring pain for gain. It says "real men" are tough guys who don't show emotion.

- **I'm the king of my castle.** It's my way or the highway. Who's the boss around here anyway? Don't I have a right to have my needs met? Being a warrior, a tough guy, a go-getter, a boss isolates a man to focus on himself. These stances reinforce the idea that life is all about oneself. The risk of losing face just reinforces the bluster. These attitudes in turn distort how a man sees his leadership role within the family.

- **Just give me a little slack.** In growing up, most of us men were nurtured with a freedom to "be boys," to engage in an acceptable wildness usually denied our sisters. Such slack is one way of steering boys toward the conventional (and superficial) view of manly behavior. Gradually as we mature, we come to expect that being given a little slack is our due. Often the person providing the slack is Mom, because Dad is too busy working or enjoying slack himself. As a result, when forming relationships of our own, we expect the same slack from our girlfriends and eventually our wives and families. Do men typically offer the same slack to their wives and children? Not usually—see the next trap.

- **You should be like me. (Or do it like I say do.)** One result of being spoiled, of being given slack, and of being expected to be tough and excel is that we men develop a sense of "our" way as the "right" way. This attitude is probably unconscious. But it sets up the standard against which we measure others, particularly our partners and children. Such an attitude is one symptom of a flawed sense of appropriate boundaries.

- **The responsibility must belong to some other guy.** Denial marches hand-in-hand with fear. If I've been taught to be tough, to stuff my feelings, and to take the lead, then if I feel vulnerable or inadequate or scared, the easiest way to deal with those feelings is to deny awareness and/or push responsibility for them off on something or someone other than myself. "*They* made me do it—I had no other choice," we rationalize to ourselves.

- **I'm too busy.** Here's another defensive move—avoidance. Taking refuge in one's busyness is another way of pushing away a sense of vulnerability and responsibility. It's also a way of refusing to look at one's feelings and the facts behind them.

- **Setting up your wife and or children for a fall. Labeling others.** This is a favorite. Have you ever come home from a hard day at work, feeling really tired, stressed and a little grumpy. All you want is your feet up in the lounger and the football game on the TV. When you hit the front door, the first thing you see is junior's soccer shoes in the middle of the hall and everybody's coats spilled all over the great room. And the hall light is burned out. Before you can think, you hear yourself yelling: "Junior, where are you? You get down here right this minute. How many times have I told you about your shoes and this mess? Can't you do anything right?" With junior scurrying, you march on into the kitchen where your wife after her long day at work is scrambling to get supper on the table. You see the white sack on the counter. "Takeout chicken again? That's twice this week. Can't you plan a little better? The only time my mother served take out was when we ordered pizza. Well, call me when it's ready."

- **Negative self talk. Negative talk about your wife or others you love.** This is first cousin to labeling and setting those you love up for a fall. In this case it's running yourself down when you don't meet your own (unrealistic) standards or running others down when they don't. It's allowing yourself to indulge in a pity party. It's holding yourself to the wrong standards or impossibly idealistic standards.

How do you get caught in negative, enabling co-dependent behavior?

If you've used the chapters earlier in this book to explore the facts behind your feelings, then you probably already have a pretty good idea of how you've been caught and where you are stuck. You may have seen the roots of some of the traps just described in your own life. If you have not used these techniques yet to explore these issues, there's no time like the present to go back and start. Use the techniques to look at what's behind your armor, to look at your relationships and ways of interacting with your wife and children, to look at what drives you.

What About Anger?

Is anger more overtly and obviously a male problem? Do men tend to explode more openly, to be more aggressive? I think, in the main, the answer is *yes*. For example, one research facilitator once asked a group of parents, "What's the only emotion that's OK for boys to have?" The answer was quick and clear: anger. This may be the reason we have so many angry boys—and men—because parents and our culture reinforce the idea that aggression, if controlled, is appropriate for men, is a mark of strength because it's emblematic of warriors and hunters, the ideal images of manly men.

In addition, this socialization meshes in potentially negative ways with the way men's brains may be wired. Substantial research has documented differences in brain structure and brain activity between boys and girls. For example, some biological differences appear to make boys more impulsive, more vulnerable to benign neglect, and less efficient classroom learners. Added to this, boys grow up under the pressure of unrealistic expectations without the balance of nurturing emotional support, so they learn to stuff and ignore emotions. The ability to feel their emotions and understand their messages without being consumed by them, an ability which would set them ahead, is lost. With that loss, boys too often then exhibit aggressiveness and hyperactivity that holds them back, that frustrates them. Boys thus combine physical aggressiveness with emotional vulnerability.

Men have both passionate and ferocious sides that can be simultaneously a source of strength and a source of weakness. Properly acknowledged, understood, and channeled, a man's passion and feelings can be used to create a well-balanced, tender, loving man who is also a dynamic (and loved) leader. Stuffed, warped and thwarted, passion and ferocity can transform into anger and hate, pushing the man beyond some ideal warrior toward "killer." In this sense boys and men slip beyond the acceptable levels of manly maleness and wildness, becoming excessively aggressive, invading the space of others in order to dominate, enjoying risk-taking activities as "really living," and asserting their will and dominance over their family and co-workers. If they thought about it, most men would not choose this way of living.

CHOICES

Claiming Your Freedom of Choice

Who are you anyway? Are you really what you do? Are you the intensity and energy expended to do your tasks? Are you the competitiveness, coolness, the anger and craftiness you exhibit in relating to others? Let's assume that beneath the competitiveness and anger and deep within your chest (if we can chisel deep enough), there lies your heart, your self with the softness and kindness you need to relate differently with others. This is perhaps the way you would prefer to be. By uncovering your heart, you can reach outside yourself and at the same time receive, listen, and communicate in a meaningful way with others. You can thus return to the real you before the armor was built. By choosing to integrate all you've learned, you can change and free yourself from the burdening falseness in your life. It's your choice, truly.

You can do it, if Jake could. Jake was the living embodiment of the aggressive, take-charge, all-capable warrior I've been describing—he could do it all and he knew it. Then came the day he had a huge heart attack, killing about half his functional heart muscle. How did he get there? Well, over 25 years, he had been so work- and achievement-oriented, that he had sacrificed his relationships with his wife, children, extended family and friends—though when asked, he'd give twenty-five excuses why he did what he had to do and ten more why it was all his ex-wife's fault. But while recovering from his heart attack, he felt ambushed and guilty. He could no longer go at his job with the intensity he'd had six months before. Yet at this slower pace, he felt like he was disappearing, like his "turf" was slipping from his control, like others would take over and his achievements would be wiped out, forgotten. He was self-centered and selfish.

But in spite of this attitude or maybe because of it, after his heart attack, Jake wanted to make some changes. He wanted to reach out and connect again with his two sons who were ten and twelve. Forced to rest and be quiet and calm, he discovered that he liked being with them. They freely offered him affection and support he didn't know he needed. In fact, he was still hiding that need from them, not really sharing the severity of his heart disease, and shifting blame to his medications for the need to go slow and for his physical impairments. He also continued to emphasize the problems and stresses he'd been under. After all, what man would want to appear weak to his sons? But these boys responded in a remarkable way to show him their understanding of what he was experiencing. One afternoon, they took him on a trek on the Internet, surfing to define *stress*. They then retreated to their den to prepare a document for their dad as seen below and presented it to him. It's a remarkably perceptive image of a broken heart.

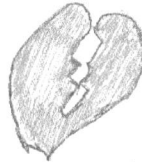

Stress can caus a broken

1. Forciby exerted influence, pressure. In dentistry, the pressure of the upper teeth against the lower mastication.

2. The sum of the biological reactions to any adverse stimulus, physical, mental, or emotional, internal or external, that tends to disturb the organisms homeostasis Should these compensating reactions be inadequate or inapropriate, they may lead to disorders. The term is also used used to refer to the Stimuli that elicit reactions.

To: Dad From: 2 ▇ and S ▇

What a thunderclap for Jake. He broke down in tears as he recounted the details. He felt overwhelmed, in a good way, in their caring for him. He felt that he appreciated his children in a new way, seeing them as real people. He was surprised that his former wife had not "poisoned" them against him, that she'd kept her complaints and bitterness between the two of them. This encounter with his sons helped Jake start to become unstuck in how he related to others, how he interacted with the world. He worked to engage his sons and others with freedom from the anger and pouting he exhibited when he felt wronged. He no longer had to keep a tough poker face and a stiff upper lip, but could respond with spontaneity and animation, enjoying and absorbing these fundamental essences of life. He felt like he began to live again.

Jake made a choice to change. Every man can.

CHOICES

You can make these choices
- as an individual
- as a husband/partner
- as a parent

What roles would you choose? What do you need to do to nurture health and well-being as well as connectedness? Here are some attributes that I've found are important concepts for men to understand.

Being gentle is not unmanly

Being gentle is a key quality for personal growth and for enabling those we love to grow. Ideally for men, the key to learning the art and skill of gentleness is to start early in life. Unfortunately, many parents (though doing the best they could) have acted as if courage or bravery and gentleness were mutually exclusive. "Be a big boy," "boys don't cry," "just tough it out, son."—you can probably dig your family's phrases out of your memory banks. Often our fathers didn't nurture this quality with example and praise. Although the gentle side of living is difficult to develop if that part of the brain is not stimulated early, gentleness can certainly be learned with practice.

The essence of this gentleness is in the ability to focus attention away from yourself and toward others you care about. Your goal is to better understand them by not letting yourself interfere and get in the way. Taking this position, you can be softer, more forgiving with less tendency to posture defensively. You'll find it easier to let the angst and anger go, too.

How do you lead in positive ways? Defining what leadership really should be for you and in your relationships.

It's an illusion to think of leadership in personal relationships in terms of being in control or in terms of the stereotype of military hierarchical command. Effective leadership in relationships is shared and is more facilitating than commanding.

The women in our lives, particularly our wives, often have an advantage in sharing responsibility and leadership in relationships because often they have learned more about the art of gentleness and communication because those values were stressed in their upbringing in ways that were not in ours as boys.

We men need to *choose* to learn these skills—or to bring them home because many of us use them daily in our work relationships. We need to *honor* our wives and children. Honor—there's another word/value that is drilled into us guys. We can put that concept to positive use. What does *true* honor in giving your family leadership look like?

Honor means looking at the "the big picture" after plenty of forethought and planning. Honor means being gentle, man! Honor means respect for the small stuff—such as your personal boundaries and those of your spouse and children. Honor means really listening and hearing—and staying flexible enough to shape your actions and response by what you learn through listening. Honor means teaching your boys early to respect women and treat them as individuals of worth, ability, and dignity equal to one's own.

You can share leadership in your family without being too rigid, without being too focused or cold. You can be warm and yet still be an adequate disciplinarian. What's the foundation for this type of leadership?

- Deep, basic love for your partner and the children you're rearing together
- Basic planning for the outcomes desired
- Coaching for yourself, through continued learning.
- Reinforcing your authority by sharing it

You can choose to be the person you desire to be for both yourself and for your wife and children. By choosing to change yourself, you can enable all to change.

Tips for giving good leadership

Remember these two important concepts:
- Leading is not commanding, it's communicating, "walking with."
- Leading is putting those you love first (spouse, children), not your "will" or pride first.

CHOICES

What Expectations Does Your Wife or Partner Really Have?

Most women probably desire some variants of these general qualities. (If you've been listening to your spouse, you may be able to give these general ideas some individual and specific twists.) Here's my list based on the experience of working with numerous individuals and couples.

What does a woman really want? She wants you
- to be there for her—to be her champion
- to respect and honor her individuality, while treasuring the connectedness between the two of you
- to be kind, trusting, and trustworthy
- to be slow to anger, blame, stand on stuffy pride
- to stay with her and never leave
- to take care of her as you take care of yourself
- to believe and behave as though she not only was once but still is and always will be perfect for you
- to convince her by your actions (more than words) that life is not about you, but about "us"
- to live and behave as though the two of you are truly a union of equal partners
- to be willing to take the first step toward reconciliation/resolution after a disagreement or fight even if you are in the right.

When I look at these, I think—and I bet you do too— "That's a pretty good list—I'll take the same." Smart man! That's exactly my point. The terrific qualities that we desire in a relationship (qualities such as these just bulleted), we can only receive if we first put them into practice ourselves.

Set your wife or partner up for gain

Usually we use the term *set up* in the sense of ensnaring someone or setting them up for a fall, but I'm using it in a totally positive sense.

Believe it! Face it. Your wife or partner will be the person you allow her to be. That person you've wanted her to be is there already, and you are the only one that can bring her out.

Do we really lose face if we aren't in charge of our "woman" or our child? Do we really lose power or authority if we give a little or compromise? No.

You can take some very simple steps that set your wife or partner up for gain. (These steps also work for your children.) Here goes:

- *Respect her time and your time together.* Share responsibility for what will happen. For example, whether you both work or not, do you touch base with her in the mid-afternoon to check when you and she will be getting home and what needs to be done for the evening to go well. When you both get home, do you focus on her for at least a moment or do you launch into whatever concerns you? Do you gladly share in making the evening go well, the household run well? (Though the vast majority of women work fulltime these days, studies show that women still do the vast majority of the chores that make a home run smoothly.)

- *Whatever happens, be okay!* If she's upset, comfort her or at least be okay yourself. Don't get upset and fussy. Don't pull on the rope even if you are irritated and the end is dangling there temptingly. Just drop it. Ask is this about me or is it about her? Life being life, stuff happens. The best strategy is to let go the need to have the last word, the need to defend your hill or your pride. Hold to the positive; let go the negative. Stay in the moment. You can be independent, strong; make it so!

- *Stay focused on her.* When you're there, be there. Listen to what may seem to be small talk to you—listen for what's important to her. So what if you think it's boring—do you think the account of your day is hot news? Pay attention to her goals and achievements. They are as important as yours, even if they are different from yours. Give her credit. Again, stay in the moment.

- *Don't put her on display.* Be proud of her but remember she isn't a trophy or a new car. She's the woman you love, that you chose to spend your life with. Value her as that person.

CHOICES

- *Talk together about what you want out of your marriage.* Really listen and update your choices. Remember that intimacy is crucial and that intimacy is at least 75% more than sex. Yep, that's right.

- *Remember you can't really control her—and you don't want to.* So just be okay. When you've hurt her, ask forgiveness and mean it. Accepting yourself and her will exude an aura of strength that's much more powerful than any show of strength that comes from defending your pride.

- *Remember how much she means to you.* Reinforce those positives.

From personal experience, I know that it can take some effort to begin to think and act in these new patterns. But from experience, I also know that it's worth it.

Yes, you take care of her and treat her as the apple of your eye with the structure outlined above: by showing more than by talking and you'll reap the rewards. You can count on that!

8

R E S P E CT — Issues for Women

In this chapter

In American culture, as in many others, growing girls are typically encouraged to strive for perfection in caring for and meeting the needs of others. As a consequence, they often neglect their own needs. This pattern holds true within marriage and family relationships and within the ways women usually approach their careers.

Like men, women's lives are filled with stress, much of which produces frustration, anger, and a sense of things being out of control. Rather than verbalize their anger, women often suppress it. But then they pay in angst or depression or in submerging themselves in everything they must accomplish. The price is loss of sense of self, lack of self-image of strength and loss of respect of others.

Women need to reclaim their strengths such as nurturing, teambuilding and perseverance and to reclaim their own self-respect. This chapter discusses how women can move the *red flags* that invite lack of respect away from themselves and claim their right to choice, freedom and wholeness. "R E S P E C T . . . find out what it means to me!"

In larger sense, more women ought to make this their personal anthem—not only demanding respect from their loved ones but giving themselves some respect.

We've already looked in Chapter 7 at some specific issues for men. In this chapter, I want to take time to look at some issues with health consequences that women must face and resolve in their relationships, particularly with men and with family.

In our society, women generally are raised and encouraged to strive for perfection in caring for others and meeting their needs. As a consequence, they often neglect their own needs. This pattern holds true within family relationships and within the ways women tend to approach their careers. Being the primary nurturing support for family (husband, children, older parents) is inconsistent with being "allowed" to be sick. As a result, many women tend to push their own health needs to the back, to neglect to take time for themselves, and to ignore the increasing toll of stress on their well-being.

Are women rewarded and treated with respect for these self-giving, tend-and-befriend behaviors? Not necessarily. Domestic violence, inequality in the workplace and at home, second-class citizenship, or even virtual bondage in some cultures are just a few realities that suggest that we've a distance to travel in human society overall.

More and more, however, many women are coming to recognize what statistics have long shown—that how one copes with life's stresses and health risk factors has an important effect on the health outcomes in one's life. For example, science has long known that heart disease is an equal opportunity problem. In real numbers, more women than men die from heart disease. Yet until recently women have not been adequately included in research. Only one woman in 28 dies of breast cancer; one in two women dies of heart disease. Yet which do you as a woman fear most? Most women fear breast cancer more.

Two-thirds of women who die suddenly from heart disease have no previous symptoms. Among people who survive heart attacks, more women, particularly older women, die in the first year after a heart attack than men. According to the American Heart Association, "Within six years after a recognized heart attack: 35 percent of women will have another heart attack, 14 percent will develop chest pain, 11 percent will have a stroke, 46 percent will be disabled with heart failure, and 6 percent will experience sudden cardiac death." We need to discuss the possibility that some of these heart disease outcomes may be rooted in how women are treated and how they see themselves personally and in relationships, particularly family relationships.

Like men, women have lives in contemporary America that are filled with stress, much of which undoubtedly produces frustration, anger and a sense of "things" being out of control. Rather than verbalize their anger or explode, women often express anger and frustration in the form of resentment, bitterness, nervous agitation, or depression. As a group within our culture, women are not reared to express or channel their negative emotions but to suppress them in support of the greater good of their spouses, families, and workplace. Yet stress fuels biological coping responses in women as it does in men. For example, physiologic studies measuring catecholamines, substances that play a role in the heart disease process, showed an increase in women late in the day correlating with increased family demands and diminished control and social support. Women's typical tend-and-befriend behavior is not consistent with setting limits and balancing one's life.

Growing Up Female in America

In spite of great strides for women (compared to 50 or 100 years ago) in education, job opportunities, and the acceptance of at least the concept that women have relatively equal status with men, our culture still operates patriarchlly, and women and men are still subtly guided toward self-concepts, behaviors and roles that diminish both women and men. For example, many women are raised with the idea that pleasing the men in their lives, starting with their fathers and transferring to their husbands, is their most important goal. As girls, women are often not offered the slack that their brothers receive or expected to be "a little wild." Instead, they are taught to continue "spoiling" the men.

Although more and more parents and society as a whole may encourage women to fulfill their capabilities in the classroom and on the sports field, for example, subtle and overt obstacles still remain. For instance, research has shown that at almost every level, teachers tend to call on boys in the classroom more frequently than girls. Each year during March Madness, I've noticed that the front page of the sports section is filled with stories of the NCAA men's basketball tournament, and even though the women's games may be just as exciting and skilled, coverage of these is buried back in the section and gets much less space. In families where both the husband and wife hold down full-time jobs and contribute jointly to the family's income, the wife typically does more of the household management and the housework.

One of the great strengths of women is that they, more than men, are nurtured to connect and to communicate. These skills and others provide strengths that women can draw on in their relationships. However, circumstances also produce behaviors that leave women stuck in unhealthy responses to stress that have negative results for their personal health and the well-being of their relationships.

Typical Strengths That Women Can Build On

Although the following qualities are strengths, I would also point out that in some cases they can be overworked or turned against women if they are not self-aware.

Ability to connect

Psychologists at UCLA studied women's coping styles and discovered that when challenged, many women did not respond with the expected "fight or flight" behavior. Instead, they sought to protect themselves by connecting, understanding (tending) and defusing (befriending) the threat. This is just one aspect of the strength of being nurtured to connect with others and to be aware of the others' needs. Of course, not all women have these skills. Or they may have twisted the skills toward less healthy ends (such as possessiveness or over-control) in a response to their life experiences.

Staying on point and being comfortable dealing with feelings

Because they are more comfortable in expressing their feelings (as I have observed in many support groups), women often have the ability to keep the group and the discussion focused on the personal issues that the group is supposed to be addressing in a given session. Where men tend to hide their feelings and fears under more superficial exchanges, once they've agreed to engage in the discussion, women typically open themselves to the risk of sharing (both feelings and facts) in order to gain the benefit. Such willingness can be a real benefit in nurturing better relationships.

Gift of "stick-to-it-ness"—perseverance

In the new grueling team sport of adventure racing, women team members are much sought after by male participants as keys to having a winning team. As reported in a recent article, having at least one woman on the team, the male participants observed, helped the whole team excel. Why? Women, said the men, had mental endurance, attention to detail and organization.

"The female presence kind of leavens the loaf. It's like a mothering thing," said one man. "I've been on races when the female thing kept testosterone from getting supercharged, where guys [would have] exploded." A woman teammate noted that regardless of gender the best "teammates in these sports are the ones who can keep themselves and everyone else going through exhaustion, terrible weather, and discouragement.... Being a mom is great training for this adventure racing: always going, doing ten things at once, and you're used to sleep deprivation. Team members have to work together, all are required to finish together, and often it's the woman who pulls everybody through."

Ability to bend

As noted earlier, under the stressful circumstances that trigger self-preservation through the built-in fight or flight response, women in many ways have transformed the "fight" or "aggressive" response into one of "tend or befriend." Most women don't need to prove that they are king (queen) of the hill and while they hate to lose in a confrontation or "difference of opinion," women are often more willing to compromise if possible or to withdraw and try again later.

Gifts for nurturing

Or as the adventure racing fellow noted, "the mothering thing."

CHOICES

Mothering skills are probably partially biological traits conditioned by upbringing and experience. Certainly, women are encouraged from girlhood forward to care for others. Playing dolls and cooking, for example, are encouraged pastimes for little girls.

Ability to put others/the team/her team first

This quality might be considered a key quality of nurturing or mothering. Just as the men in the adventure racing team praised the positive benefit received from their female member's ability to do what was best for the team as a whole, so many individuals would recognize this ability as part of their mother's contribution to the Family.

Typical Ways Women Get Stuck in Stressful Behavior That Has Health and Well-Being Consequences

Do you ever find yourself playing any of these scenes?

- **"Mothering" as "spoiling"** used as primary mode of relating to husbands and children can trap women in bribing positive reinforcement for themselves from those they love. Certainly, mothers want to support and nurture their children just because they love them and want what's best for them, but when "support" becomes "indulgence," important boundaries are violated.

- **Oh, me? I'm fine.** When confronted by being made the butt of a joke, verbal aggression or even being taken for granted, many women stuff their feelings, rather than constructively express them. Stuffing feelings of hurt eventually leads to resentment and seething anger with the problems that brings (see Chapter 6).

- **Poor little, defenseless me.** Even when a woman has suffered the brunt of anger or verbal abuse, taking refuge in victimhood is a trap. Victims don't have to take responsibility for their own actions; they can lay their inaction on the aggressor. Victims can also continue to poke and prod at the aggressor— baiting that individual so that the victim can use "victim status" to continue to excuse their inaction.

- **I can't help it—that's just the way I am.** Describing a choice as immutable fate is a very specific form of negatively labeling oneself. If you are trapped by past experience and your "nature," then you are convinced there's nothing you can do to make matters better. This trap is a way of avoiding your responsibility for the matters that are inside your own sphere of influence. It's also a negative way of coping with unwarranted or excessive criticism from one's spouse; such a trap tacitly grants approval of the spouse's negative opinion rather than asserting quietly one's own integrity and individuality.

- **Negative self talk.** Many women verbally run themselves down; they may even cast this in tones of charming self-deprecation. However, such negative self talk produces labels that you live down to. It also lets you off the hook of being responsible for yourself.

- **Labeling the other as a way of exerting control.** This trap is often a natural reaction to having felt put down or victimized, particularly when you've buried the resentment for a while before you explode. It's so easy to call names—and at first that may seem so satisfying. But labeling is a dead end. It's particularly a dead end if you get stuck in seeing the one you love as you've labeled them and don't allow them room to change.

- **The children come first.** After children arrive in the family, some women relegate their partners to secondary status. This is a huge trap. The health and security of the children rest first on the identity of a couple as a "we." Parents together may make sacrifices for their children and that can be wonderful—as long as the sacrifice is not your partner and the vitality of your relationship with each other.

Specific Issues Women Must Address to Build Better Health and Stronger Relationships

For many years, my wife and I have worked with numerous women who faced the challenges of coping with stress, improving their health and creating more satisfying relationships.

CHOICES

We've concluded that women frequently face situations that undermine their freedoms. These circumstances generally spring from cultural concepts of women's proper roles and duties, then are reinforced and/or adapted by specific family patterns. Let's look at several.

- **Losing your identity in the "service of others."** Many women accept the idea that their first duty is to serve others, particularly their husbands and families. At its most extreme, this view holds that submerging themselves in the care of others is "what women are put on earth for."

  Although dedication to service can be a worthy value, when service requires denying and confining one's gifts, graces, and self, what's going on is "being used," not true service. And it's not healthy for women or their families. Such self-abnegating "service" frequently results in giving others, particularly men, too much slack for behaviors that violate boundaries or are otherwise selfish or abusive. This way of relating does nothing to foster clarity or communication between partners or good parenting and nurturing for your children.

- **Accepting subservience to men.** When women buy into flawed ideas of service that require self-abnegation rather than self-fulfillment, they also typically become trapped in subservience and submission to the men in their lives, first their fathers, then boyfriends and husbands, and finally even children, particularly sons. But giving up your identity in this way is stressful and unhealthy. You suffer the consequences and so does your spouse and family. The family needs you to be yourself—an individual who knows how to express her goals, dreams, concerns, a co-leader with your partner, and a role model of a whole person. If you are enslaved to meeting others' needs, you are not only unable to make positive choices for your own well-being, you are not able to really nurture them and influence them for positive ends. Healthy relationships require equal partners, whole persons, not "masters" and "servants."

- **Giving others, particularly your spouse, too much slack.** From the time they are toddlers, as I've discussed, boys and men enjoy extra leniency. They are expected to be a little wild and to violate the boundaries—"just being boys." As boys mature, typical patterns of child-rearing continue to indulge boys in this wildness and to spoil them. As a consequence, many men as adults and husbands expect the service and the spoiling to continue. If you give the slack and the service, even when your spouse ignores or violates boundaries, if you act to placate, appease, and please when he is indulging in inappropriate behaviors, then you are doing your husband and yourself no favors. You may think of him as independent and yourself as bound, but he is just as trapped. Rather than being independent, the spoiled male is dependent on being served. He's usually downright demanding. And it wears you out, right? The more you'll give to appease and please, the more he'll take. And the less respect you will receive, the less recognition of your personhood. Becoming a martyr is not a healthy woman's goal.

What To Do?

Break out and be yourself—take back the slack

Withholding slack helps you help yourself by keeping others in check. Respecting yourself fosters their respect for you and ultimately their self-respect. (Less guilt.) You hold on to that slack because you are a person of value. You uphold values that are important to you and reflect them in the life you lead. Using your understanding of your past experience, you are now clear about the appropriate boundaries you wish to maintain; you are clear that others must be accountable for themselves. If you are not giving your slack away daily in "spoiling," then it's a meaningful gift of true service when you share it in appropriate circumstances. So *keep your slack intact* for the right occasions.

Claim your leadership role

Did you know that you're the most powerful and influential person in the whole wide world—the family world? "If you ain't 'happy,' then nobody's gonna be happy!" But it's important to remember that your spouse isn't necessarily trained in making you happy. He's looking after his self-centered, spoiled self. Your task is to encourage him, not chide him, and to continue his training as you continue your training. Yes, you are able to do it—it's in your nurturing side —if you do it from the start. You have to insist that the two of you minimize all you both have learned and start your relationship afresh. It's imperative to your survival as a united couple.

You can make him a better family leader with you by ensuring that you have a voice in your partnership –making certain that the two of you are united and that you make decisions before the need to execute them arises. Together with your spouse you need to practice sharing your views and making decisions together. You must also claim your role as co-leader in the family. Most women, after all, are the parent who is most frequently in the trenches day in and day out.

You can claim your appropriate leadership role only by making changes in your own behaviors, by modeling the strong independent woman you want to be. That means taking responsibility for yourself—no falling into the old traps, or at least climbing out of them as fast as possible.

Don't think you'll be able to love your man into change; that approach simply doesn't work. Love him because you love him; treat him like the man you expect him to be, but don't set about trying to change him. The only person you can change is yourself. You can change to be the person you truly want to be. Then you must continue to be that person for yourself. Forming a win-win relationship begins with being true to yourself, then consistent and communicative with others. Such an attitude—remember you are staying within yourself not trying overtly to change the other—can also have a transformative impact on your partner.

Give yourself the right to freedom and change

This point is at the heart of what I've been talking about in claiming your independent self and leadership role. You must apply it in all areas of life. Be true to yourself. Keep working for self-actualization. Stand up for yourself: Don't take putdowns from those closest to you or as far away as media images (ads, news, movies, etc.). Let go the hurts and failures. Encourage your daughters and other women.

Changing after we are adults is not as easy as when we were younger, but remember we human beings are plastic—biologically and psychologically—and can change. Many old messages from society and from your family, though they are irrational for today, still exert their influence. Everyone still responds with the old automated reactions we've internalized. So give yourself permission to claim the freedom to change.

Find the help you need

Standing up for yourself isn't easy. There will be disappointments and failures. But we should take to heart the example of the unsinkable Molly Brown as portrayed in the musical about her. Mrs. Brown was real-life Colorado pioneer who survived many adventures and disasters including the sinking of the Titanic. After multiple financial disasters, Molly was asked why she persevered. Her answer: "Nobody wants me down like I wants me up!" A winning attitude.

But for most of us a winning attitude isn't quite enough. Many women have not been raised with the tools or building blocks they need for self-nurturing. And reading this book, or several, isn't enough help. At this point, you may wish to reach out for additional training and resources. For example, classes in assertiveness training, communication skills, or negotiation management can be helpful.

Support groups can be wonderful—and they may not look like what you think of as a support group. One friend of mine enjoys her long-time bookclub—sure they discuss the book but the personal sharing and support is just as important. Other friends have found support in yoga, martial arts, or dance classes, in extended education classes (or going back to college), or in church activities and study classes. And there's the Red Hat Society and other similar groups. Finally, I've seen such support provided over and over in rehab support groups after physical illness.

If you have been in an abusive relationship, finding professional help may also be a very positive step toward claiming your life for yourself.

CHOICES
Moving the red flag away from your heart

In losing their identity in so-called service to others, many women hold a metaphorical *red flag* that attracts attack (like the bullfighter's red cape) right in front of their hearts and bodies. Such stress not only takes an emotional toll, it takes a physical toll. By looking at your history (the messages you've been taught and labels received), by examining your strengths and traps, by claiming the vision and resources you need to change, you can move the red flag away from your core being. This gives you the freedom to see more clearly (is this about me or them?) and to make the changes you desire.

Reminders Going Forward

For you

- Show respect for yourself
- Be yourself at all times
- Create time for yourself
- Nurture yourself
- Build a support network
- Stay connected with other women
- Rise above your past thoughts and emotions to pursue your goals
- Remain flexible
- Continue to redefine relationships with meaningfulness
- Develop positive self talk—focus on a positive authentic you
- Become the leader you were meant to be
- Avoid the victim role—you are responsible for you
- Never accept negative labels and don't deliver any

For your children

- Treat, view, and mold your children as you desire each to become
- Help your boys be responsible and sensitive to you and others at least as much as pursuing their wild side

- Support your girls as you would boys

For others, including your male counterpart

- Put your professional feet forward in caring for others: maintain distance and establish boundaries

- When serving others, understand whether there is a trade-off and/or an end in sight

- Get educated about life with men, first from a distance

- Talk with and listen to the experiences of other women in your network

- From the first encounter, avoid giving a male any slack

- To be worthy of a relationship, a man must put you first and show his commitment and responsibility through his behavior

9

How to Get Unstuck—Using Personal Experience, Behavior, and Values as Keys for Growth

In this chapter

What does it take to make the changes in life that you wish to make? It takes a journey, not a single decision or choice. Getting stuck along the way is a given, even if you start smoothly.

This chapter provides techniques that function as strategic guides to keep your feet on the path. They help you see the real you that you know deep inside that you are and that you may have "protected" or "hidden." You'll learn step-by-step and day-by-day that you're able to intentionally be and share this real you with others.

The strategies help you identify your bedrock values, accept yourself and others as persons of value, and learn to let go old baggage. They help you better process and progress through hidden or hurtful issues, not dwell on them. With your growth will come new vision, purpose and potentials.

When we begin to explore our feelings as guides to the facts behind our present choices and actions, we must first acknowledge that we are stuck. Sometimes it's almost as if we were up against one of those force fields in science fiction—you can't see it, but you sure know it's there. To be stuck is to be caught in reactivity, rather than to be able to choose your response.

Maybe you haven't used the word "stuck" to yourself, but unless you are reading this book under threat of something more powerful than your own resistance, you have already acknowledged that something needs changing and that you are ready to try.

What Does It Take to Make the Changes in Life You Wish To?

In my experience, you've got to recognize and use two realities:

1. Acknowledge the ways in which you are stuck, the ways in which habit and fear of change keep you from achieving the growth and peace you want.

2. Look to the facts you discovered (and will keep discovering) using the techniques of Chapters 5 and 6 as the beginning of an exciting journey that leads to your goals, that leads to freeing yourself from the restraints and recycled responses that keep you from *being*, and enjoying, your true self. And remember at every stage—whatever the stage—there's hope.

Personal change requires a journey, not a single epiphany

As you explored your feelings and your past using the techniques in Chapter 5, you probably had a number of "a-ha" moments. With each experience explored, you probably felt that you were learning more and more about some of the facts that have influenced the way you live your life today. Those insights alone can feel like a fresh breeze blowing through a stuffy room. But a quick caution: remember that insight rarely produces instant achievement. The insight is absolutely necessary, but achieving the change takes you on a working journey—a journey, for most of us, on which all our personal naysayers try to discourage us along the way. They often yell loudest not long after you start.

Personal change requires looking at the facts first from your perspective, then from the perspective of others

To make personal change, you need to step outside yourself mentally to see yourself as separate from encounters with others. Rather than focus on the painful feelings evoked by memories of hurts and griefs, you must look at these as objects or factors in a story that has meaning for you. As an actor on your own stage, how do you come across to yourself?

In addition, personal change requires seeing ourselves (as best we can) from the perspective of others. Their words and actions reveal perceptions that have something to say about how you or your behavior is being perceived. Just as you looked at the messages present in the stories and relationships of your growing up, you also need to look at what the messages are in current relationships. What do these have to say about yourself or how you are coming across? Be careful not to jump to judgment, especially if some of the perceptions sting. Grant the other individuals the same wishes, desires, and obstacles that you have. Here again using the Johari's window diagram can help you think through these different aspects.

Claim Your Personal Power And Equipment For The Journey Toward Change

An ancient Chinese proverb says that the journey of a thousand miles starts with a single step. Personal growth is also a journey. The seven steps bulleted here will help you along your journey. Notice that each point starts with an action verb. Why? Because the more you practice each action, the more each is transformed into a power-ful vehicle or tool to carry you toward your goals.

1. Identify your personal values. These are your individual bed-rock.
2. Accept yourself as a person of value.
3. Respect the dignity and individual "personhood" of others (particularly those in close relationship to you and those who were your "teachers").
4. Learn to let go. Letting go means forgiving yourself and others as well as letting go the hurts and griefs of past experiences.
5. Stay open to help from others.
6. Embrace life as an adventure. (Or at least, be comfortable with life as an adventure.)
7. Be yourself at all times.

Now let's look what constitutes each step.

Step 1: Identify your personal values

Your personal values are the bedrock of who you are—your personal identity. Choices in life—both conscious and unconscious—stem from personal values. In turn the outcomes of those choices continually reshape values. With positive choices you can shape positive values that work for you, not against you.

Using the exercises of Chapter 5, you identified a number of the messages and labels that you have received in life as well as the values that you learned through those messages and by other means. If you have not already done so, it's time to think deeply about those values.

- Which values are still appropriate for your life today and which are not? What new values would be more appropriate? Why?

- Think about the role your values play in the relationships you have with others. What do you value in relationships? How would any new, more appropriate values you've identified enhance these relationships?

- What boundaries are important to you? Boundaries also help define who you are. Have them clearly in your mind, both for yourself (what you are free to do and what are your healthy inhibitions) and for others (how they relate to your space). What do your boundary definitions say about your values?

To keep your focus in the shifting shoals of life, your goals for growth may seem more concrete if you actually write down both the *keepers* (the positive values you want to build on) and the *blockers* (the negative values that have been holding you back and that you want to let go).

Also note why each value is important or problematic. It may help to identify the most significant memories and feelings associated with each value.

Use your identified values as touchstones as you continue to work on your goals.

CHOICES
Step 2: Accept yourself as a person of value

Accepting yourself first means rejecting the old messages and labels that keep you stuck in feelings and behaviors you no longer choose. Rejecting these messages doesn't mean rejecting the messengers or teachers. Instead, you simply take back the power you've given them to make your choices for you.

Accepting yourself means being okay with yourself. Each of us is wounded from life. Be comforted: you are not alone. Accepting yourself as worthy frees you from constantly trying to prove worthiness with selfish behavior that keeps shouting "I'm the center of my universe."

As you are okay with yourself, you can relax to grow and change. You can listen easily to others, without getting defensive. You can let go your lapses and failures.

For me as a person of faith, accepting myself as a person of value is grounded in my relationship to God and my understanding of God's grace, a free gift of love that accepts me and every human being just where we are and just as we are. Whatever your faith tradition, acknowledging support from your spiritual Higher Power can give you tremendous freedom. Accepting that I, like every other person, have infinite worth that allows me to be me and you to be you.

Along the journey when you experience hard times, frustrations, doldrums and setbacks, remember: This too shall pass. And nothing can change my worthiness.

Step 3: Respect the dignity and individual personhood of others

This step follows naturally from step 2. If I'm okay, I can let you be okay. Just as you have seen the dangers of labeling for your own life, so projecting labels onto other people is a way of trying to control them. What we say about others often says more about us than it does about them. For example, if someone constantly applies negative labels (jerks, idiots, butts, ignoramuses, and worse) to persons whose actions displease the speaker, what does that tell you about the person who uses the labels? What if they just "think" the labels? Don't we usually see fears and defenses coming out in that name calling?

Blaming someone else, cutting others "down to size," or belittling the value of any other person sends you down a dead end road. Maturity grows when you respect, value and honor other individuals. This is critical for those people close to you. For instance, it is natural to want to blame those who may have taught the messages or values you have found most destructive. But don't go there. Remember they, like you, were just doing the best they could at the time with the understanding and resources they had. It's hard, however, not to blame unless you take the next step.

Step 4: Learn to Let Go

If you look at the seven steps as a mountain climb, then learning to let go takes you to the top-most peak. You have to climb hard to get there, but after you reach the top, it's downhill the rest of the way. Although learning to let go is a continuous process because old habits and mindsets die hard, grasping the essentials takes only a moment of recognition.

Letting go requires three choices:

- **Forgive yourself.** Remember you are a person of value. You may be sorry (or angry) for what you felt you let happen to yourself, sorry for things you have done that hurt others, or weighed down by the angst of personal burdens. Forgive yourself. Remember you are worthy. Use the lessons from the past, and set your feet on the journey forward.

- **Forgive others.** The reasons for forgiving yourself also hold true for other people. Forgiveness may be hardest to extend to those you care most about—parents, children, life partners, best friends, close colleagues—but these are the persons for *your* sake that you most need to forgive. Respect and honor their dignity and personhood. Remember that they usually were (and still are) doing the best they can with the understanding at their command.

    We need to let others be themselves, just as we need to be ourselves. That means we need to let go the notion that we can change anybody other than ourselves. You may find it helps to imagine your sphere of influence as a clear

Plexiglas cylinder of a diameter that extends only to the fingertips of your outstretched arms. We can be of help to others, bless them and allow them to be okay, but we can't change them or remake them in our idea of what they should be. We can respect their individuality, honor their independent selves, and allow them freedom to develop into the persons they want to be. You can only change what's inside your cylinder.

- **Release the hurts and griefs of the past.** History has value when you learn from it and move on. Get beyond the old stories. Throw out the baggage of the past. Let go the old, worn-out working models. Understand them, use them, then let them go. Letting go helps you to stop drawing defensive lines in the sand on every issue. Letting go frees you to build on the positives. Letting go helps you to deal with anger, to express it appropriately so that you use it as a springboard for growth, rather than a torch for setting a destructive bonfire. Letting go frees you up to be you—and to reflect on events maturely, to be okay and open with others, to share yourself, to create happiness and new memories, and to discover deeper meaning to life.

Learning to let go can be of particular importance in your quest for healing and health if you have heart disease, cancer or another serious illness.

Remember: Letting go isn't a one-time thing. It's a process, or tool, with many elements (such as reframing, relabeling, changing heart, changing attitudes, growing) that you'll use over and over for the rest of your life. Practice may not make your ability to let go perfect, but it'll sure make it easier. Each time you feel yourself holding tightly to a hurt, ask yourself if that hurt's worthy dying for. What are you making the investment for anyway? After a while, I promise that you'll wonder how you ever lived without the powerful tool of letting go.

Step 5: Stay open to help from others

Letting go within yourself is not the total answer, for you must also give the problem(s) to someone else and be open to feedback about how well you are doing.

Trying all by oneself to overcome many hurts and griefs, to cast aside worn-out messages, and to choose new behaviors is a lot like trying to fight an aggressive bacterial infection without antibiotics. As the fever rages, false messages of defeat and rejection feed on isolation. So don't even try to go it alone. Gratefully accept the presence of help. This is a spiritual response that goes beyond biological, physiological and psychological issues. In my experience, the most effective place to share it is with your Higher Power. Whether that Higher Power is God or has some other meaning for you, giving your griefs away to that accepting reality usually works better than sharing with a fellow human being. Does that mean you should not work with a therapist or share with an appropriate friend. No, those experiences can be very valuable and are often appropriate and necessary. But sometimes we have to open ourselves first in secret to our Highest Power before we can truly trust others—and accept the risk that they may not prove trustworthy.

You may, in fact, have to give the hurts and griefs away multiple times, for you may have concealed their roots in many areas of your life and the hurts may resurface several times. Such recurrence is not a defeat for you but a victory, similar to climbing stairs one step at a time. Usually letting go is easier the second time and beyond. With victories, your grip on your emotions, your anger, your pride may seem stronger but will weaken as you insist on your choices for change. This process opens the door to your heart and softens it again so that you can be more accepting of change, which makes it more likely to last.

Accurate feedback about oneself comes only from others. If you have done your primary work, including stepping outside to look at yourself from your perspective and then from the perspective of others as we talked about earlier, then you know that there are some things you can't do. For example, you can't give yourself accurate feedback about whether or not what you intend and feel as sincerity and genuineness is being received as such by others. That insight can come only from observing their responses.

So as you go forward with relationships, you can be okay whatever happens. You can listen and not be offended by anything. You can say thanks for information and then evaluate it. Even if you judge that their feedback is wrong or skewed, at the very least their reactions and responses tell you something about them. You need all that information for your journey. I would note that this same attitude is helpful when faced with illness.

Step 6: Embrace life as adventure

Or at least get comfortable with that approach. Sometimes we may dream of living in some paradise away from it all. Yet even as we fantasize about such a world, we know it will never be. Life for most of us is more like swimming or paddling a boat on a lively river. Upstream or down, the river is filled with challenges. Or think of some other adventure image that fits you better. Whatever adventure image you chose, you can't live life worried about all the things you can't control. Instead, you must focus on what you can learn and experience that will enrich life and your relationships with others.

Living life as an adventure requires living in the moment. Not the past. Not the future. Just the now. Living in the moment requires honing the crucial ability to focus and refocus on what's important as the adventure unfolds. I like to use the image of docking a boat because, like life, accomplishing this seemingly simple task requires handling various forces that make reaching the goal—safe harbor—harder than apparent.

Some forces are in my control—such as my ability to handle the boat skillfully and maintain it so that there is little chance the engine will stall at the wrong time. Other forces are outside my control but must be constantly observed and taken into account—such as the direction and strength of wind and current. So as I back the boat in toward the dock (and between two other boats), I must focus and refocus on my goal. I have to keep my eye on a point on the bobbing stern of the boat and another on the edge of the dock as I slowly and gently guide them together. I have to sense the effect of the current and wind and adjust steering and engine power to keep on target. You can imagine all the little adjustments I have to make to reach my goal—docking the boat—safely and smoothly.

Certain abilities can help me accomplish this goal. First, I have to stay relaxed and welcome the challenge. If I get tense and rattled, simple things become hard. I have to have confidence in my skill and knowledge of my limitations. It's freeing to acknowledge the fact that even with my boating skills what I'm achieving is essentially a controlled crash. Next, I have to shut out other concerns as distractions—a healthy denial—and live in the moment, focusing and refocusing on docking as forces involved in the task shift. Third, I have to be ready to adapt and try a different way if something, say a rough chop and stiff crosswind, blocks my first approach. All these skills are elements of enjoying life as an adventure by living in the moment.

Step 7: Be yourself at all times

When you've practiced the first six steps, you'll find it easier to be the person you want to be, perhaps even the person you have always been inside your armor. You can stop being somebody you're not. Up to this point, perhaps you have been more comfortable changing hats, wearing a different one for each task and occasion, perhaps being a different person in each different context and relationship. You don't need to live like that. You can be the same person for all tasks and occasions. You are capable of achieving that goal.

To achieve that goal, however, you'll need to bring your whole self and your skills and capabilities to each relationship, task and setting. It took me a while to learn how to do that and how rewarding it was to be my full functional self whatever the occasion or place.

During my transition years I was not a model participant. As a physician I spent long hours at work focused on serving others and helping them deal with tough health problems, sometimes devastating illnesses. I put my whole heart and energy into caring for patients, and without thinking too much about it, I received maximal support from staff in my practice. It was easy to carry the concerns and burdens of work over into family time. The first thing I learned was that it was okay to leave work concerns behind, physically and mentally, when I left the office.

But I was still the center of my universe. I was so used to the support of staff at work that when I got home I silently demanded my right to have even more support there. That support took the form of my being catered to and relieved of responsibility for the quality of family life. Silly me, I even expected my wife to do all the work for both of us—the thinking, creating, initiating, the follow-through and the working both on our personal relationship and the quality of family life. It took me a while to see how selfish and spoiled I was acting.

I finally realized that although I was comfortable using my people skills at work (listening, observing, understanding, not being defensive or taking comments personally, focusing and refocusing, living in the moment), I was not bringing these skills home or using them in my personal life. I also realized that, like so many other guys, I thought I had to get out of the house, away into the woods, out on the water, or on the golf course to find myself, to relax and be myself. Then one day when I was having a great day with my family, was feeling and being completely myself, I saw the light. I said to myself, "I can do this—be myself—here and everywhere. I can incorporate my supportive people skills into my natural way of living because they help me share the real me."

With that insight (years in the making), I was able to extend myself to others at home as well as at the office and not have my energy sucked from me. What I had been doing before was more fractured, took more energy, and was less rewarding than being my full self and using my skills and gifts in every relationship and activity.

This insight also meant that I finally granted myself adult status equal to others—I didn't have a particular place that I had to fit into. As a result, I no longer gave power to their messages and labels or reacted unthinkingly. Instead, I was able to see and be myself without qualifications. At work, one small outcome of that choice was that I began to treat even older mentoring physicians as colleagues, including calling them by their first names (with respect) as they had always called me. With my family of origin it meant that I quit reacting to fit handed-down messages and labels. Instead I shared my real whole self with them. I took my turn at child care, at cleaning up and doing the small stuff. When I went to the amusement park or ball game with the kids, I relaxed and took my whole self (I left the dictation at the office).

Most important, I no longer took encounters so personally. I didn't have to defend every thought or comment when challenged by others because I realized that the subject was not always about me. I ceased to see everything from the "me mode," and those general tensions that permeate our lives eased. I also saw that life was about focusing and refocusing in another sense. Just as a bullfighter uses the red cape to draw the bull's focus away from himself, by refocusing I have moved the red flag away from my heart so that other people's actions and statements are no longer personal assaults or provocations to defend myself.

Don't Give Away Your Power to Defenders of the Status Quo—How to Recognize the Negative Forces That Fight to Keep You Stuck

No matter how ready you are for personal growth, no matter how clear and simple the seven steps seem, the journey inevitably has a few potholes and roadblocks. I call these blocking forces your *personal naysayers*. Everybody has them. Some come from within ourselves; others lie outside ourselves. All these naysayers defend the status quo—they want to keep things just as they are. Recognizing the characteristics of some of the most common can help you move beyond them.

Cloaked resentment. If you are not honest about your hurts and griefs but keep the feelings stuffed down, then you are likely to keep the anger at what's been done to you stuffed down. Such hidden resentment tends to turn our focus to "what's wrong with them" rather than "what can I do to help myself."

Avoidance, or *hiding*. As you've been reading this book, have you caught yourself saying, "that's too much trouble," "I'm too busy to do that," "that's not my problem," "that'll be too upsetting," or making similar objections? Such thoughts are clues that you're running away or hiding from the process. Fear is usually behind avoidance—fear that what you discover will hurt, fear that you'll lose control, fear that you'll lose your sense of who you are, and so on. Once you acknowledge and name that fear, you can move beyond it. You always have the power to choose unless you give it away.

"Defending my hill"—stubborn denial. Do you take everything personally? Do you find yourself defending your position on every issue or explaining actions (even if nobody asked)? Does every attempt at a serious discussion with a spouse, child or parent end up in an argument? If you find yourself continually defending your hill, explaining everything, or issuing ultimatums, then you are stuck in denial. This naysayer is kin to cloaked resentment and fear, and like them, tends to shift the focus away from what you can change—yourself—and toward what you can't change directly— other folks. Stubborn pride usually means placing the blame on others rather than understanding the facts, letting go, and going forward.

"I'll try. . ." This naysayer builds in an escape hatch from the first. It's a first cousin to the naysayer *avoidance,* and like avoidance it also stems from fear. You'll remember Master Yoda in Star Wars teaches Luke Skywalker the importance of committed thinking: "Do or don't do!" Yoda says, "Forget try."

Fear of losing the "Self" I'm accustomed to. It's always hard to leave the known to journey into the unknown looking for a new world. But remember, you are always you, you are in control, you make the choices.

Fear of failure—the change I achieve won't be better than what I have now. That's always a risk. But that unlikely outcome would still leave you no worse off, so what have you got to lose by choosing the journey? As reassurance, I can say that in my many years of helping others undertake the journey, only a handful of people haven't made what they felt was progress. And that handful were those who refused to risk the journey at all.

Other people. Family and friends—particularly if they love you dearly, often get used to you the way you are, plus they have their own issues, fears and defenders of the status quo. Many in your circle of family and friends—even your life partner—may not have the desire for change at the same rate you've chosen. Or they may see your changes as criticism of them. Remember in this case that it's okay to be the new person you've chosen to be. Be tolerant of their differences and resistance; don't take it personally as rejection. Also avoid attempts to change them. Later they may appreciate your changes and growth and desire to join you. Let negative feelings toward them go and keep the door open. Keeping the door open doesn't mean you put yourself in a position to be beat on continually, just that you stay available to their potential for growth and change.

Resistance from those you love may also simply be testing behavior. If they hold hurts and griefs associated with you, they may wish to be sure that you've "really changed" before they trust you. On the other hand, if they have not been working on self examination and growth themselves, they very well may keep labeling you and shoving the same old baggage in your direction. Don't take it. Be okay, not angry, not defensive even if you have to withdraw from the hostility. Remember if you stay okay, slowly they will change, too, in their own time. You'll learn there is more power in your being okay than in trying directly to change them.

The Payoff—The Value Of All This Work

After you've experienced choosing new directions, letting go, and letting others help, then you can say you did it. You took the problem from the thinking stage of a nebulous, swirling, upsetting energy of thoughts and transformed them into concrete reality. You no longer have to listen to the programmed messages in your head. You got your thoughts, feelings and messages out, became vulnerable, risked letting others hear them and opened yourself and your needs to others. You loosened your grip on your problems, your head messages, your anger, your pride and gave them away, thus you softened your heart. You also released the physical burdens that exact a health cost.

Using this chapter with chapters 5 and 6, you can begin the journey to becoming the person you want to be, living the fulfilling life you choose. As you work with these chapters, you may find the following *Tools for Insight and Change* give you more resources to organize your work. Chapter 10 then shares some reflections on using your spiritual resources. Chapter 11 provides some specific "relational" tools that will help you do a better job of communicating your thoughts and goals to yourself and to those with whom you share relationships.

MORE TOOLS FOR INSIGHT AND CHANGE

Chapters 5, 6, and 9 provided some specific exercises to enable you to explore your personal history, to identify what's really going on under your feelings. The tools in these chapters may be sufficient or perhaps you'd like a more specific outline for working on issues. That's the purpose of the tools in this section. First, I've provided a week's worth of daily exercises—the pattern you can use for study each week—whether you set your own topics or use my suggestions. The second tool is a 36-week calendar of weekly topics for study that you can use as a springboard for your work. You should also feel free to rearrange the topics I've outlined or add to or subtract from them. Also don't forget to allow an occasional week for rest and "down time." Always remember: *slow* is Good.

Since one size (or order) of schedule does NOT fit all, I've provided on the website a blank 52-week 'calendar' that you can use to map out your own topics and progress. Feel free to draw from the topics on my calendar as you create yours or ignore it all together.

A STRUCTURED WEEK OF EXERCISES

You can use this pattern of work with any topic as you work toward positive change

Day 1   Define my issues on the topic. What is it? (or several "its") Lay the issues out. No judging, just defining.

Day 2   Focus on an issue or two. Dig deep. Explore. Look for similar stories that reflect the same issues, behaviors.

Day 3   Dissect what's going on. How do you feel about it? How do you understand it? What's positive? What's not? Why?

Day 4   Evaluate the feelings and behaviors related to the issues for your earlier circumstances and for NOW. Which work positively? Which don't? How would you choose to change?

Day 5   What will you act on? What choices and behaviors will you "update"? What will you let go? What do you wish to affirm and build on?

Day 6   Play/Family Day

Day 7   Rest/Family Day

A CALENDAR FOR REFLECTION, CHOICE AND GROWTH

Remember that this calendar is just a suggested order. You may rearrange, expand, subtract and otherwise shift the topics to fit your needs.
Also remember to build in some weeks off for rest and family fun.

Part 1: Exploring Self and Roots

You may wish to explore these general topics using the "storytelling"
technique by picking appropriate springboards (p. 93) or creating springboards to get you started.

Week 1	Who am I?
Week 2	What are my roots? Childhood?
	Interactions with mother? Father? Grandparents? Others?
Week 3	What are the important messages I learned in childhood? Adolescence?
Week 4	What's my image of my present life?
Week 5	What are my main sources of conflict? Where are the roots of the conflicts?
	What are the messages and beliefs fueling them?
Week 6	Conflicts continued (if need be)

Part 2: Exploring Self and Relationships

Week 7	What relationships are important to me?
Week 8	Reality versus fantasy in relationships.
	What reality in relationships is important to me?
	What is really fantasy or "if only"?
Week 9	Relationship with spouse or partner
Week 10	Relationship with mother and father.
	What are you taking with you forever?
Week 11	Relationship with child or children
Week 12	Relationship with friends. Why did you choose these friends? Do they encourage you to leave your "ruts" or to stay "stuck"?
Week 13	Relationships with co-workers. What are the personal dynamics of your workplace?
Week 14	What do my relationships say about me?
	What aspects of how I relate work?
	What would I choose to change? What would I choose to let go?
Week 15	Pick a relationship, then ask: What is my sphere of influence? How do I use it?
	What about boundaries? Do I label and button push or support positively?
Week 16	What can I change about me to make me happier and bring out the behaviors I desire/cherish in another?

The work of the first sixteen weeks provides all the raw material you
need to explore the topics in the following sections that can help you

"peel back the layers" of experience. So dig back into that material as you work on these specific "angles" and choose behaviors that you desire (both to keep and to change).

Part 3: Exploring feelings and behaviors

Week 17   Overall, am I optimistic or pessimistic (a grump)? What experiences or issues fuel my general outlook and attitude?

Week 18   What makes me really angry? What are the roots? Can I give up or let go something without anger or being defensive? See Chapter 6 for specific help with anger.

Week 19   What labels and messages shape my feelings and choices? What are my "buttons"?

Week 20   Do I have clarity of thought and emotion? Have I learned that emotions can be positive cues that lead to facts? (Think about this question particularly in the context of your personal life and relationships.)

Week 21   What is my world view? What are its roots? What do I affirm in it? What would I change? If I am having trouble letting go, why am I staying invested in something I see as negative? How can I understand and choose differently?

Week 22   How many hats do I wear? What are they? How can I wear one hat? Plan and implement one change this week to help you reach the goal.

Part 4: Envisioning and choosing for the future

Week 23   What do I value most in life? What do I wish for in my life? For myself? For my family?

Week 24   What will I and my life look like in five years? Ten? Twenty?

Week 25   What will I need to do, to choose, to change to reach my envisioned life? Plan a small step to take this week to help start toward my goal.

Week 26   What will I need to let go to enact my choices effectively? Plan a small step to take this week.

Week 27   Can I live one day at a time? Can I live "in the moment"?

Week 28   Can I live without guilt? Can I let that go? Can I let go anger and choose other responses?

Part 5: Communicating

Week 29   Can I get quiet and listen to what I'm feeling and thinking inside? Can I be okay with that? What's my "self-talk"?

Week 30   Am I connecting? With myself? With spouse/partner/ family? With others?

Week 31	Am I listening? Paying attention to feelings—mine and others—and then shifting to the facts? In all relationships?
Week 32	Do I choose my words? Am I focused on the larger picture? Am I labeling?
Week 33	Can I be assertive without being hostile and defensive? Can I use "I" statements effectively? (Have I actually practiced it?)
Week 34	Am I connecting with my spiritual side?

Part 6: Your choice

Week 35	Identify an issue I feel still needs work
Week 36	Review steps I've designed or chosen to help me go forward. Make a brief but clear plan for progress.

Part 7: Blank calendar form for creating your own work plan

To create your own work plan you can make a table or spreadsheet on your computer, or use a notebook.

10

The Spiritual Power of Choice

In this chapter

Freedom grows from connection not isolation. Each person desires to be wholly oneself. But you cannot be wholly *you* until you decide to complete the connections in your life by letting go the bonds that bind your spirit.

Letting go old baggage and old ideas, letting go defensive walls frees the vital spirit within to connect. The power of choice lies in the unhindered freedom of the chooser:

- freedom from self-centeredness and selfishness
- freedom from reactive stances rooted in personal past history
- freedom from the need to control
- freedom from distractions blocking connections with others and
- freedom from distractions or forces obstructing one's relationship with God

Spirituality is about selflessness—about connecting deeper within ourselves and beyond self with others and with God. It's about relationships that paradoxically free us to be wholly and completely ourselves. Such spiritual connection ensures a peace, an improved tolerance to illness if it's inevitable, an improved mental outlook, and fewer precursors to disease formation. This chapter explores practical ways to tap the spiritual power of the freedom to choose.

The Spiritual Power of Choice

Once, many years ago in an eastern land, a man was out walking when he looked up and saw a tiger staring right at him. Instinctively, he began to run away from the danger. Suddenly the edge of a cliff loomed. Looking back over his shoulder, he saw the tiger charging straight at him.

Without thinking, he jumped off the cliff. As he fell, he grabbed a hanging vine. As he hung there, happiness at his luck flooded his being. As he drew a breath of relief, however, scraping, scratching sounds reached his ears and vibrated through the vine. His gaze jerked upwards.

A rat gnawed at the anchoring end of the vine. He looked far down to the ground below and then up again at the rat. Down at the ground, up at the rat, his heart hammering in his chest. Down, up; down, up. Then, he saw it. Right in front of him appeared the most beautiful ripe strawberry he'd ever seen—his all time favorite fruit. Cautiously, he balanced himself, foot against rock, and reached out, picked the strawberry and ate it. It was delicious—absolutely perfect.

What's the point of this mystical little tale? The man made a choice. Confronted by danger and stress before and after, above and below him, he could have continued to panic and to scramble. Instead, he stilled himself in the moment, accepting the reality of his situation but open to perceiving the moment of pure beauty and perfection right before him. He had no other way out. Neither skill, nor busyness, nor scrambling (and certainly not desire or prestige or power) could rescue him. So he acted from his heart, in the moment, without regard to his past or future. He made the most of the moment. The story ends there. But who is to say whether or not the man's being in the moment and staying open to both fact and possibility without anger or panic might not have opened some other avenue as perfect as the strawberry?

We each desire freedom to live life to the fullest. That freedom comes from our desire to shed the baggage that binds us to our past and predicts our future. To do so takes us to our core: our identity, to the foundations of our beliefs. Our identity allows us to release our past burdens, protective armor, and future fears, to enjoy life where we find ourselves, and to enjoy what's right in front of us: the "strawberry." In so doing, we don't keep our minds on the tiger, the rat, or the impending fall, for they only bind us and blind us from seeing the strawberry. Once we are able to see the strawberry, we are free. We are then able to connect from our hearts and capable of experiencing life to the fullest.

It's no accident that at its core the story of the strawberry is about spiritual power. The concepts I've been discussing in this book go to the center of our identities as human beings. The power you possess to look to your feelings as guides to the facts of your relationships is a spiritual power in important ways. We human beings are complex creatures—a wonderful interweaving of biology, psychology, intelligence, and spirituality. You can be a person of deep religious faith or no religious faith and still affirm this reality of human existence. From research and experience, I am convinced that our human power to choose is a profoundly spiritual reality that we can draw strength from.

Recently, I was reminded of an observation made by C.S. Lewis, a widely read and influential twentieth-century Christian layman: "Evil is always man's doing, yet it is never his destiny. The power of choice makes evil possible but it's also 'the only thing that makes possible any love or goodness or joy worth having'." There's freedom and awesome power in the ability to choose. The power of choice lies in the unhindered freedom of the chooser:

- freedom from self-centeredness and selfishness
- freedom from reactive stances rooted in personal past history
- freedom from the need to control
- freedom from distractions blocking connections with others
- freedom from distractions or forces obstructing one's view of God.

Our spiritual side, then, is all about moving away from self to connect with other human spirits and to connect with God. Spirituality is about selflessness—about connecting deeper within ourselves and beyond self with others. It's about relationships that paradoxically free us to be wholly and completely ourselves. Such spiritual connection ensures a peace, an improved tolerance to illness if it's inevitable, an improved mental outlook and fewer precursors to disease formation.

When I look into the eyes of a loved one, I realize that I'm looking at Love itself and am awed. Staring into those eyes, I peer into the depths of the person and through them into the eyes of God's pure love where I am accepted unconditionally. What I see is the power of that Love. And reflected in the eyes of this Love I see my own eyes. Love is a universal fullness that's transferred from person to person; through our imperfect love we connect and yearn for the more perfect connection with God.

The wonderful thing is that each of us can, of our own free will, choose to reach out beyond the "me" mode and connect. Such free choice is awesome, exhilarating, and in its purest state, it's the simple, positive side of free will—without the burden of the layered, encrusted, historic, personal negatives.

But there are many blocks to exercising this deep spiritual power of choice. Although my Christian faith is vital to my life and I will be sharing from that foundation in this chapter, the definition of spirituality that I'm using is broad enough to include many approaches to faith. I want us to look particularly at the selfishness, pride and greed that lead to deceit, lies, and self-centeredness.

The discussion of the first nine chapters of the book leads to the conclusion that humankind's free will is not usually free. That's a tough idea to swallow after you first realize it, isn't it? Your will is especially not free when you remain trapped in "forced to react" mode as we've discussed. Each day in any situation or connection, our free will to choose confronts a fork in the road. One path leads to "what I must have for me." The other path leads to "what I desire for you and what I can do for you."

But the opportunities for change abound—opportunities for meaningful, healthy, long-range and permanent change. Being able to choose change, however, requires being "OK" and accepting yourself where you are. No matter how broken you may feel you are, no matter how much something inside cries out to blame something or someone for your state, choosing to change means first accepting and understanding what has been—the past—without blaming others or yourself.

The ability to do this is for me the gift of God's grace. Grace is a gift of acceptance that you don't have to earn; it's yours just because you are a human being, a part of God's creation. God's grace is manifest in our ability to change. It makes healing possible.

It's a part of our being, we only need to engage it by recognizing our connection. Even when we know God provides healing and the miracle of repair for us, we still tend to reject the gift because the burdensome baggage of our past interferes.

I find it immensely hopeful that almost weekly new data from scientific research confirms that change is a natural part of our make-up. Our body tissues, organs such as the blood vessels, heart and brain can alter themselves towards recovery in response to an insult. The brain, for instance, contains the capacity for certain parts, under certain situations, to become "plastic," which is a capacity to restructure to recover function. This is relatively new information. This is the way we were made.

These new discoveries reveal marvelous processes. Most of us know someone who, with great effort and determination, has overcome some tremendous obstacles after an accident or severe illness to regain their physical and mental abilities. Mental, psychological, and spiritual aspects of our being are integrally and powerfully connected with the physical aspects of our being. These connections can serve as supports or obstacles.

We are all aware of times in our lives when it was easier to accept, adapt, or learn something that was too hard to tackle previously. It also is obvious to many that there are common milestones in our lives when it's easier to change. It's as if there's a design built-in for change. Something changes inside, a softness appears, perhaps unexpectedly, and, at that moment, we're ready. Change enters through portals. Portals open during these softening periods of life, letting in the opportunity for change. Portals are pathways through which we connect with others: physical, mental, psychological, and spiritual pathways. These connections are necessary pieces that make us complete. We are truly works in progress.

What Does It Take to Change, to Forge New Traits?

First and foremost is the power of a spiritual conversion experience. Forging new traits implies we change from the inside-out, essentially changing our character, and such change always requires help from beyond ourselves. Although change must happen inside, sometimes the process may start from the outside and work inward as when one practices a certain discipline (such as doing the exercises of Chapter 5 or the practice of daily prayer or meditation) until it becomes internalized.

The process of forging new traits has different components and proceeds through stages. First, it's about you, your "self," and your patterns of discipline (placed there by others). Then, it's about others. It does not work without opening yourself to the spiritual power that is greater than your individual self. For me, that power is the presence of God's grace and love. For you, that grounding may take a different form, yet it is there whether you are aware of it or not. (If you want to be amazed at the interconnectedness of all life, just read some of many studies on the importance of the balance nature requires for health in almost any ecosystem.)

Unless we are able to accept ourselves and circumstances as they are and then to let them go so that we can listen and grow, we will continue always processing the next word and action from the other person or anticipating their thoughts, moves and motives. The purpose of such processing is to maintain the status quo, to avoid change, to defend ourselves and our turf. At that point we are usually unable to see our own motivations in perspective even though we are mired in thinking of ourselves. Being so focused on self and self protection makes us blind to others. We're then unable even to hear any thank-you's—if they come—and can't respond with a simple "you're welcome" for we are unable to hear and listen to what the other is saying.

No matter how many self-protective actions we take, they can never provide fulfillment in life. Instead, we just add more layers to our armor. We may never get beyond this layered armor unless we understand the full influence and power of choice—both choice we make consciously and choice that is automated behavior. Our true maturity, which includes hope and vision, leads and enables us to reach beyond ourselves to others—it enables us to place our experiences within a bigger picture. We can separate ourselves and our experiences from those of others. We can choose to be okay. We choose to let go control where it is counterproductive.

Focusing our minds and becoming still (prayer and meditation are two long-proven techniques) set us up to be receptive, to be comforted by the quiet, to let the loud distractions fade out into silence, to hear beyond the noise of self. At this point we tap the ability to self-nurture in empowering ways. For me, this quiet centeredness opens the door to communing with God, the relationship that opens up to me the opportunity of achieving my full potential. As a Christian, I believe that God is not "out there" but here with us and within us, the sustainer of life. This faith image expresses the ultimate "belonging" or "at homeness" that I believe every human being has in the universe. We are all connected—and across every division you can think of. To affirm this image is to acknowledge that even when we are alone we are never isolated and it can empower us to choose to reach out to relate to others.

Opening up to the spiritual power to choose moves us beyond living a life bound by "do-s" and "don'ts" to a life enriched by grace—amazing grace that affirms that you are worthy, that you have value and dignity and the ability to choose to make your life new is empowering. Such grace is also the road to peace:

- Peace with yourself
- Peace with family—parents, siblings, children
- Peace with problems
- Peace with health
- Peace with life, filled with thankfulness and forgiveness
- Peace with loss of life, with death
- Peace with your place in the Universe, with your Higher Power, with God

Within the context we've discussed, the following techniques and tips may help you tap into the spiritual power of choice.

Mastering a New Outlook

As I've said so many times throughout this book, you are on a journey to a new way of living. Mastering the new outlook needed is not one-and-done, but a continuing process. It takes practice to get comfortable with the new approach outlined in Chapter 9. The exercises of Chapters 5 and 6 helped you begin to use some of the techniques that can help you create the portals for change and free yourself to choose. These are a great start to developing the skills that make a new outlook second nature—something you don't have to stop and think about. Here are two simple techniques that I think can help you channel what you are learning and open new vistas as you continue on your journey.

Weekly time for me

Make an appointment with yourself for a specific time each week—a half hour or hour—for reflection. I suggest that you get out of the house—perhaps a walk, or a cup of coffee at your favorite coffee shop, or a quiet seat in a garden or park or beside a stream. (The nineteenth-century American writer Nathaniel Hawthorne said he did some of his best thinking during lengthy sermons on a Sunday morning.) Use this time for affirmation, reflection, and renewal.

- Affirm and be reassured that:
    - I'm not alone—I am a part of the Universe; God is alive in me—family and friends who care for me are available
    - I'm forgiven—I can let go stuff that happened to me and places where I feel I've failed; I can choose to be OK, then go about my life
    - I can choose to live in the moment and to act in ways that help me reach the goals I've identified
    - I can follow the good health practices that support my journey (eating right, exercise, practicing relaxation/stress-reducing techniques, complying with my meds)

- Reflect on the week just past and even further back as useful:
    - What actions and choices do I affirm?
    - What do I need to let go? What mental clutter? Negative messages? Guilt? Busyness? Obsessions?
    - What one or two things will I work on this week? Next week?

- Renew affirmations and commitments
    - To live in the moment
    - To let the past go

CHOICES

- o To keep going forward
- o To take one day at a time
- o To let go negative self talk and to affirm the journey

Journaling

Write it down. Write it down. Write it down. Keeping a journal doesn't need to be fancy, stylish, or grammatical. But writing your thoughts down—just for you—does at least three things:
1) You get your thoughts and feelings out—it's a way of not stuffing them down.
2) You don't lose those thoughts, feelings, insights— particularly when they are negative. Sometimes we stuff the things that anger and hurt us the most because we are afraid of losing them. Journaling helps you record the negative—so you can let it go—and remember the positive—so you can build on that power.
3) By reviewing your entries over time, you can observe your growth, make course corrections, and be thankful.

Preparing and Living Out Each Day

Each day presents a new opportunity to make new choices, to live out the day the way you wish. Here are three techniques that I use to help me live in the moment and choose to be my whole self in every encounter and relationship:

Wake up call

As the day begins take ten minutes to rehearse what you want to accomplish in the day and how you want to interact with others and the day's challenges. After your ten minutes, forget it and just get on with the day. The ten minutes could be shower or shaving time or even your morning run/walk/exercise time. I know some busy parents who get up ten or fifteen minutes before anyone else just to have this "quiet time." Some things I typically review or remind myself of include:

- o I claim distance on the me-mode.
- o As I listen to myself each day, I will hear and learn the negative messages I was taught and cull-out the unwanted and/or irrational ones for today.
- o I will give each person with whom I interact my full attention in the moment. I rehearse listening and giving clear responses, other communication skills.
- o As the day progresses, I quit practicing and use all I have in the moment to be a win-win encounter.

Take a time out if needed

This is a tried-and-true stress relief technique. When/if the day ratchets up the tension—or maybe it's just one stressful encounter or demand—give yourself a quick timeout. It could be in the office or at lunch or a break. Shut off or ignore the phone. Sit quietly, push all thoughts out of your head, focus on a quiet mental image if that helps (sunset, rippling stream, clear blank surface) or focus on your breathing and heart rate, thinking slow and quiet, relaxing each muscle starting with your toes and progressing to your head. If thoughts drift in, push them gently away but focus on the breathing and relaxation. Give yourself ten minutes. Then start the rest of the day as if it were the first of the day.

Defuse a tense situation by intentionally examining what's really going on in it—not just reacting

With a little practice, using the following questions or a shortened version of them will become second nature even in the heat of the moment. It will help you choose your response rather than simply reacting, no matter how hot or conflicted the situation is.

- Who's in control?
- Is this about them or me?
- Am I connecting?
- Do I have clarity of thought and emotions?
- Am I focusing on my own issues—keeping my "peepers on my own paper"?
- Am I living in the moment—attending to each person and/or task?

CHOICES

- Do I know, understand and own what I'm saying?
- Am I explaining too much?
- Is this the battle I'm to fight?
- Do I understand the problem?
- Is this the time to let it go?
- Have I uncovered all my options and choices?
- Am I attending to life's rules rather than being thankful as I interact with others?
- Am I doing more talking or walking?
- Am I being OK?
- Am I being?

What is the strawberry for me now, at this moment?

What gift is there for you at any given moment, if you look for it? We are often too busy or too afraid or too something-else to stop and open our eyes to look for it.

A friend and patient of mine, Fred was once a driven but very successful man. Yet a severe heart attack gave him an opportunity to change. If anything, Fred is more successful now but he's also happy and at peace in a way that's never been true before in his life, in spite of the real health issues he must face daily. What's his strawberry? "I am continually looking for ways to make a contribution that will have a positive impact on the quality of other peoples' lives," said Fred. For him that has made all the difference for his life.

CROSSOVER to FREEDOM
through the OVERFLOW

The integration of choices, health and disease, and quality of life

The Problems

Though we appear as simple beings, we're quite complex. A lot goes on beneath the surface and, as is said, still waters run deep.

Generalized Response to Stress—Basis for Disease

When challenged physically or emotionally, humans are hard-wired to defend themselves. Challenges are stressful and threatening. Defenses respond to real or perceived stresses by assigning an immediate assessment: "I can conquer," "I'd better run," or "I'm had." In each case, the assessment stage generates an adrenalin-laden fear response: fight, freeze, give-up or run away. The emotional challenges usually involve relational issues that effect heart and mind and contribute to welling up of defenses and/or internal desires. Threats produce anxiety, fear and anger. Our brains hold the capacity to mute or reverse the reactions, giving us more control and choice.

Our pasts are filled with learned lessons that have conditioned us how to respond, certainly many from positive lessons and some from negative ones. With some, we're exposed to both. When less mature, under stressful circumstances and fueled by anger, we often follow the more negative choices, reacting with hard headedness and tending to act-out against our best interests. These reactions can create negative self-concepts, including learned guilt and thinking others don't understand or care, contributing to isolation and helplessness. It makes it hard to do the right thing or follow the rules we were taught.

CHOICES
Stress Begets More Stress

These reactions, whether toward others or toward ourselves, can produce physiological changes of which we're not aware. The sum total of the abnormal reactions is astronomical. The actual stresses in the brain and body are greater than imagined. The imbalanced neurohormones affect neurons and their support structures, even to the expense of altering the neurons themselves. Both brain and body begin changing early in the disease timeline. From the outset, genetic gateways are turned on and extend even beyond the offending agents' influence.

Familial Influences Add to Stress—
The Need to Know Yourself

Greater stresses may be beyond our control, but ongoing, subtle behaviors, especially those passed down through family generations can have considerable damaging impact on the development of self-talk, habits, reactiveness and disease. These things can be changed. Continuing to pass the destructive behaviors from parent to children is not in the children's or our best interest. In knowing this, we have an obligation to become aware and change. Our future is at stake. We need to become informed about who we are, the way we are, why we've become this way, and chose to change.

Behaviors as products of thoughts, feelings and beliefs contribute to thinking, choices and actions and all determine who we are. Behaviors encompass attitudes and their manifestations. Representative behaviors include a) comparing ourselves with others; b) the critiques that flash through our minds as we observe others, even those we don't know; c) the degrees of competitiveness we display in our own minds and with others, whether they know it or not; d) viewing self as more important than others, staying in the "me" mode; e) the non-constructive grumbling without solutions; f) the glass half-empty view of life; g) the extreme search for pleasures in socially acceptable areas, the habit of which becomes out of control, thus controlling the individual rather than controlling it; and h) the desire for what we don't have, in the pursuit of "having" or happiness. (These last two pursuits can degenerate into an alternate form of worship). And these are just a few possible responsive behaviors. Of course, there are also the standard defenses listed in psychology texts (listed as abnormal defenses), as well as in texts from all religious resources (resources for instructions in how to live). That these texts are so numerous and the best selling books in the world suggests the importance of these issues.

Couples Beginning a New Life have Stress

Imagine the added stresses contributing to a marriage because of the coming together of families with differing cultures. The process of building a relationship might be difficult enough from their beginning. Small wonder couples have conflicts after the children arrive. Parenting children, money matters, sexual issues, religion and politics provide rich opportunity for conflict for all couples.

Fostering Diseases

The problem encompasses and integrates all that we are, our whole being, including our health and relationships. Compensations and inflammatory reactions I've discussed continue, unhealthy behavioral choices are made and isolation and even depression begin. Thus, in both mind and body, negative processes begin, the basis for disease formation.

The Solution

I've always thought of the ingredients of my own makeup, in descending order, as physical, intellectual, emotional and then a little spiritual. Now, after experiencing life, I view the order as the reverse and mostly spiritual. These ingredients are more than compartments, they are hierarchical tools with spiritual at the top. It matters, because without increased awareness of the tools available, we'll not continue to grow and develop or find purpose in how to use them. Living life is all about behaviors, identifying the unwanted ones and how to influence the growth and integration of the preferred and healthier, more spiritual ones for our benefit. Stresses will persist, but our reaction to them is what's changeable.

CHOICES
Spirituality, God and Gifts

More than we realize, behaviors and much of life are spiritual matters. We categorize subjects in our minds, possibly to avoid ownership. We frequently maintain separateness between spiritual matters and our belief systems, but are they really separable? Our thoughts, feelings, behaviors, choices, both internal and external reactions and intentioned actions for many are spiritual. Of course, some of these issues are also sociological. They tug at our neighborliness, expose our humanity, and challenge our sense of community. These are the issues that test us beyond self and our ability to engage and connect with others, especially to those we may not personally know. They encourage us to reach out to others.

All these issues relate to something greater, lead us to reach further, such as to the universe that connects and integrates us all or to a higher power. For the Jews, Muslims and Christians this is the God of the Abrahamic religions; while, for the Hindus, it is the Brahman. In all cases the believer is made more powerful through his or her faith. They all relate to something greater or to a higher power. Belief systems are gifts.

Are Gifts to Be Earned?
What Was the Parents' Role?

Rather than accepting a gift with thanks, we act to earn the gift. The need to earn and repay are integral parts of our lives. These learned lessons are taught to us by those who were also taught, down through generations. Does this behavior correlate in any way with spiritual issues that may interfere with our belief system? Yes, for it originates with the God-surrogates, our parents and authority figures all important to us when we were small. Many people report to me that they hate their parents but love God. They voice no other issues or risk factors, but discussions suggest uneasiness and unhealthy moods and habits. Often their blood pressure is high. Might this suggest unresolved issues needing to be addressed? As children, we are also taught "Do what I say do" (parental verbal instructions), but more often mimic parent's habits and actions. When children are manipulated to do the right thing, rules can become hard to tolerate. The adult struggle is with rigidly learned rules that take on a worship-like fervor (fill-in your own list of examples).

Continuing in the Struggle—

Life is More Tolerable after Integrating the Gifts
What Is One to Do?

Living life and maintaining focus on what's in front of us, on the present, gives a quality gained only by living in the moment. The quality of such a life would be freer if reinforced by clear mindedness, clarity of thought and emotion, discipline and self-control. Further changes, made possible through the gifts, can lead to other spiritual issues like acceptance of yourself, in addition to feeling connected to your parents and to God. For acceptance of yourself is, down-deep, dependent on acceptance of parents, whatever they did or you perceive they did to you. This acceptance is dependent upon letting go. Sure, in all things, acknowledge your anger and fears, write them down and review the appropriate chapters in this book to put it concretely on paper. Once on paper and out of your mind, it stirs up less chaos and fewer confusing emotions. (You don't have to share what you've written with your parents and, in fact, it's better not to.)

Problems can loom in your head even after a parent has died, leaving you feeling in need of liberation. The exercises in this book will help you let go the "baggage" you harbor deep inside you. Another place to begin is to grant yourself the right to leapfrog over the burdens drowning you. Release both those burdens and tensions so you can relax and feel the calm for a change. After a rest in this "holding position," you may spiritually reconnect and move forward because you're now freed. Freeing yourself from your parental burdens opens you to free yourself of more layers of defenses and again reconnect at a deeper level with your higher power, with family, friends and those around you with whom you desire more meaningful relationships.

Incorporating Eastern Thought

Western thought focuses on the ego with the self as the basis of personality. Psychiatry has long focused on building up the ego through "self" in therapy. The West takes its thinking along when moving eastward; however, Eastern thought has penetrated western culture. The emphasis turns away from the ego and self to beyond self and on to others. Non-self Eastern thinking is spiritual and religious. Moving beyond self through meditation is therapeutic. Meditation is akin to prayer. Both are calming and give health benefits. The essence of the concept is to let go the self, to open oneself to be a part of something greater, and to include others. Thus, by focusing within, and knowing self with a selfless, non-me-mode focus, one can make the change within, accept and respect self to finally escape self and become open to others. This process opens one to the service of others and is found to enhance the freeing process. These are more spiritual gifts.

Finding Freedom—
Preparing for the Rest of Your Life

It's clear that whatever belief you follow, however you resolve your stresses, and however healthy you are, life will continue to be challenging, even a struggle. The solution is viewing most human issues as more spiritual. It's at this level that these gifts serve as sources of strength. These gifts enable one to let go, give in and be freed from the burdens inherent in the struggle. While learning more about yourself can be a gift in itself, another gift is repeated in the spiritual realm, by accepting the gift of the spiritual freedom it brings. It's without cost and something you can't earn. It's something you can only appreciate and be thankful for. It's something you can put to use. It can be the resource for your strength for life and meaningful change.

- Choose Freedom
- Change
- Enhance Your Choices
- Accept the Gifts
- Live Through Overflow

Such change produces better choices. As more thoughtful choices bring changes in heart and mind, life takes on new meaning. Reactions to stress change and you become free to crossover to accept self as a worthy being, to release life's many learned burdens, to let go of self, and to reach out to others with genuine, authentic and heartfelt behaviors.

What's achieved brings a new beginning for better health and relationships. It's also as though the "spiritual-related" change isn't as costly as change with a stressful struggle and it may well enhance the process of healing. With your belief, faith, knowing yourself, living in the moment, having clear mindedness, clarity of thought and emotion, discerning when issues are about you versus the other, and fortified with the tools of discipline and self-control, your freedom is protected, and you are provided with the strengths needed. You'll then be able to choose to become free of your burdens and be free to continue in the struggles life's journey presents. Without needs for all the armor, your true self can emerge. This is at the center of who you are. With your freedom, you'll have true freewill and be free to live life to the fullest: you can simply be. Since your gifts will be an integral part of you, you will live through the overflow of who you are.

11

Living in Relationships—The Circle of Life

Practical Techniques for Listening, Talking, Sharing, and Growing in Relationships

In this chapter

Although life events and external circumstances can be tough, the most challenging stresses in life involve people, either the ones you live with or work with or those from your past still living in your head. In the first explorations guided by *CHOICES*, you've been exploring your own depths and experiences. This chapter addresses ways to explore and achieve your goals in important adult relationships. I particularly address relationships with your spouse, but this chapter's techniques for communicating more effectively are also appropriate for relationships with friends, parents or adult children, and co-workers.

Most of us go through life *reacting*, even when we think we are *responding*. When we react, we are not really free to respond to the other person. When we react, we are giving that person power over us. Being able to respond grows out of three important techniques that enhance relationships:

- **Listening**—hearing and understanding the other person
- **Talking**—communicating your meaning clearly and in ways that the other person can hear
- **Thinking**—reflecting on what you've learned in order to continue going forward

This chapter shares practical techniques for each of the three communication and growth keys.

When I saw the *Lion King* with my grandchildren, I was struck by the vivid rendering of the idea of the Circle of Life. This reality of the interrelationship of life, one we instinctively recognize, lies at the heart of this chapter. Although you and I are unique individuals, both of us like other human beings live in relationship with other individuals and the community. Even hermits and lone wolves who eventually isolate themselves from human contact, don't grow up and mature in a vacuum.

Whatever the nature of specific relationships—from close connections to family, friends and coworkers to distant links to the hundreds of unknown people we pass on the highway or share the planet with–we need tools to help us communicate as clearly as possible. I think every human has three broad categories of relationship to address, and each takes separate (sometimes overlapping) communication techniques. Those categories can be defined as our relationship with ourselves with other people, and with God. Just as Chapters 4 and 5 have helped you explore your relationship with self and Chapter 10 looked at spiritual relationships, communication with others is the focus of this chapter. Although the techniques can be adapted to use with a wide range of relationships (from children to strangers), our discussion will focus on adult relationships, particularly those with persons you are close to.

Achieving Personal Goals in Relationships

As you discovered in earlier chapters, as you used your own feelings as clues to the facts underlying experience and memory, the task of understanding what's going on is complex because so many factors are intermixed. Adding your complexity to that of another person in a relationship just creates an even greater tangle, doesn't it? You may be familiar, for instance, with the observation that marriage involves at least six people, not just two—you and me and both sets of parents. Yes, we recognize the truth in that concept while we laugh at the humor in it. Too bad we can't keep laughing as light-heartedly in the midst of keeping real relationships afloat. But that's the point I want to make: with some insights, a few tools and some practice, you can let go and stay in the moment to achieve better communication and thus help build more satisfying relationships.

CHOICES

In the previous sections of this book, I discussed the importance of learning to identify and let go past hurts in order to choose your responses to stressful situations rather than simply react as programmed by past experiences. I also introduced the tool of the Johari's window to help you visualize areas where you needed to become more "transparent" and less governed by stuff you were unaware of. But in real-life's swirl of daily activities and interactions, it's easy to fall into behaving in ways we wouldn't choose if we could sit down and think about it. In spite of what we've learned about ourselves, we find ourselves seemingly compelled to react. Once again our relationships suffer.

Before I provide some specific tools for better communicating in relationships, I'm going to share a story and a tool I call the *Dynamic Scale of Polarized Reactivity* that offers one way to make sense of that daily tangle of perceptions, coping mechanisms, adaptations, and emotional energies that affect relationships.

Falling once more into the fray

Dana and Don were sitting in chairs opposite each other in their counselor's office. "I hate you!" Dana caught herself in the middle of her exclamation, then continued, "This is crazy because at the same time, I know I love you! Which is it? What's going on? I'm confused. So let me start over, the facts in my head and heart tell me I love you, but I know I don't like you right now." She was as upset as she had ever been in the two years since she and Don married. Through counseling, she had discovered that she tended to build up resentments, perhaps a natural trait for an exhausted pleaser. She'd realized too that this was a pattern reinforced by growing up in the midst of conflicts between her now-divorced parents.

Don understood that situation, he felt, because his parents had always engaged in loud, hurtful bickering. He had always wanted to rescue his mom and had vowed to treat his wife better, but, to his bewilderment, a strange and powerful force overtook him when disagreements or problems arose between him and Dana. At that moment in the counselor's office, he was stonewalling Dana, wasn't talking much, wasn't hearing a word she was saying—perhaps his mind was on the business trip he was about to take. Abruptly he said, "Have you noticed—we seem to need to 'fight' every time I leave on a business trip. It's like a weekly ritual."

178

Dana nodded, adding, "it's almost like we have to fight in order to part. We don't seem able to stop reacting this way."

"That's one thing I can agree with," Don said. "It's like we are forced to react."

Though Dana and Don had both done a lot of work on what was going on behind their behaviors, they were having lots of trouble using those insights to develop better communication and better ways of interacting with each other. Everything seemed a big confusing whirl of emotion and reactivity. How could they love and hate each other at the same time? How could they want to reach out to each other and then slam the doors every time? Both of them thought they longed for a little peace, but then each got upset if the other withdrew. What was going on?

The Dynamic Scale of Polarized Reactivity

Sorting ourselves out and choosing to respond rather than react is not easy when so many conflicting attitudes and feelings exist simultaneously. For example, Dana wonders how she can love and hate Don all at the same time, but she has not yet realized that the aspect of his behavior that's most hurtful, that bothers her the most, is the way he seems to withdraw and tune her out when she gets upset. Taking a look at the *Dynamic Scale of Polarized Reactivity* might help her to understand the interrelated dynamics affecting their communication.

Dynamic Scale of Polarized Reactivity

POSITIVE FACE - open to seeing self accurately

Love - Warm - Happy- Open - Freedom - Friendly

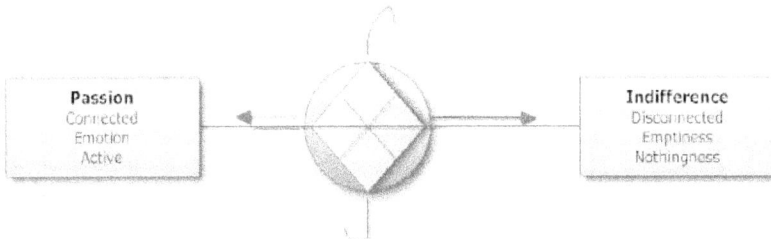

Passion		Indifference
Connected		Disconnected
Emotion		Emptiness
Active		Nothingness

Hate - Cold - Angry - Closed - Bound - Hostile

NEGATIVE FACE - closed to seeing self accurately

CHOICES

Typically, we think opposite sides of the same coin—they are opposing faces of an active, passionate emotion. Their true and deadly opposite is indifference—the total lack of caring. You can identify other active, passionate emotions that are opposite faces of the same coin. It's easy to see how these emotions can swing rapidly between negative and positive. But as long as a person is actively engaged, then a door of opportunity is open for understanding and change. It's when feeling and emotion slip toward indifference that the greatest danger of losing the relationship emerges. With many active emotional issues, opinions may unexpectedly change by 180 degrees depending on the persuasive powers and facts presented.

Each of these opposing emotions carry weighted feelings. Out of anger, resentment and hate, for example, grow the perception that one's not respected as an equal. So one begins to demand expected "rights." If the other person rebuffs these desires, that rejection may trigger seething anger and recurring hurts. These accumulate, creating gaping wounds that progressively kill hope and unleash indifference. As the indifference sets in, frustration and despair move in and paralyze any action. Despair erodes hope through inaction and the door to illness is opened. At this point, there's still a chance to act: if a trickle of hope remains, the door remains open and one is able to act. Through an open door, the injury can receive nurturing attention and the healing process can begin. Eventually, the 'indifference' will be transformed faster as the agonizing wounds heal, supported by good communication that conquers the ever-cautious fear. Perhaps the fear initially serves to protect the wounded, providing safe harbor in order for healing to take place. Then, if the individual is comforted and supported, trust and acceptance will be restored and hope enabled.

To make such change and reversal possible, you must have good communication skills and have a degree of clarity of thoughts and emotions. In a moment I will share a number of techniques, each of which helps you be "okay" so that you can focus on the task at hand and not be stuck in "forced to react" mode. So before reading the techniques you might take a moment to use the Reactivity Scale to help you focus on the tasks.

Look closely at yourself as you stand deep in your hardships, facing your problems with or in a specific relationship (or relationships in general). Ask yourself these questions:

- Can I attend to the tasks at hand, not take them to heart, and not personalize them? Or do I take them to heart, personalize them, get lost in them by grabbing the bait to explain, justify and defend my position and myself?
- If I'm not free to be the person I want to be, am I forced to react, thus bound by my emotions, distracting me from the task, binding me to my past? Using the scale, look at some of the emotional places where you may be stuck.
- Do I get the point that I need desperately to change and respond the way I truly desire to?
- Can I deal with the issues from my nuclear family and others in my past? Aren't those issues mostly in my head? Am I stuck? Am I forced to react, to re-create something out of my past, or am I simply stubborn, insisting on my ways?
- Do I understand that I can better change others by first changing myself?
- Can I be OK with myself?

Being OK is the key to using most of the following communication techniques. Being OK in this way will perk-up your antennae and heighten your sensitivities to the other person. Your goal is to know the other person's hope and pain, to take their view, see what they see and accept them as they grow. This includes holding back judgments, criticisms and corrections. To be OK is to accept yourself and others, be available, listen, focus upon the other and their issues. If you're OK, you'll be able to better keep things in perspective, view situations from a distance and process the best options as their choices are thought through.

Being OK is key to the insights that will help you respond rather than react. Being OK is the key to good communication and to freedom.

Here's another perspective on reactivity from Jeff VanVonderen.

Reactive people have not learned how freeing it is to respond to someone's behavior. Healthy responses are based upon what is true, what is beneficial, and what is appropriate. People who are not free react in order to control the situation. When your sense of well-being comes from the performance of another, you are assigning that person a lot of power over you. Their words and behavior have power to indict or vindicate. The other person has the power to establish your self-esteem or to destroy it. Therefore, control or be controlled.

Pretending to go along with things on the outside that you don't support on the inside is not submission, nor is it humility. It is dishonesty —and probably a spiritualized sugar-coating over seething anger, as well. Giving up your own dreams, your ideas, your very identity in order to earn the approval of another is not submission, nor is it real spirituality. It is a tragedy. Living this way will make you sick.

From *Families Where Grace is in Place*

Used with permission.

Getting Down to Business—Techniques and Tools for Communication and Growing

Personal growth and growing in relationships is a lifetime process. Likewise these techniques for communication and growth are not "one and done." They are life skills you can use from now on. The more you put them to work, the more they'll become second nature. The more you'll adapt them to your individual situation, the more effective they'll grow.

In his book *The Art of Helping in the 21st Century*, Dr. Robert R. Carkhuff, a noted expert in the psychology of human relations, observes that in any encounter with another person we can choose to take one of three actions—flee, fight or relate. Of course, "relating" is what we want to do with others.

The techniques in this chapter enable you to do better at three activities essential to building and nurturing relationships:

- **Listening** (Hearing and understanding the Other)
- **Talking** (Communicating your meaning)
- **Thinking** (Reflecting on what you've learned in order to continue going forward)

Techniques for Listening

Effective listening has three goals:
- **To hear/observe the content and feeling** of what the other person is saying and
- **To understand** what they are trying to communicate and
- **To acknowledge** to them that you hear and understand.

The following techniques may seem simple, but they really work because they help you practice what's often called "active" listening.

Be there! Listen in the moment. Give the speaker 100% of your attention. Let go distractions for the moment. No daydreaming or mental wandering. No anticipating the next item on your agenda or the next thing you have to do. Resist the urge to formulate an answer (or defense) to whatever the speaker is saying.

Several actions can reinforce the fact that you're listening—both to the speaker and yourself:

- Make eye contact.
- Face the person, even lean toward (alert physical posture, not slouching)
- Relax. Resist fidgeting, flipping through the paper, reading a magazine.

Focus on understanding the other person's content and underlying emotion not on your reaction to it and what you'll say about it. Your objective is to hear and clarify the other person's message, not to begin talking as soon as you can about what's on your mind. Avoid offering unsolicited advice or holding yourself up as an example.

Listen with an open heart and head. Be open to *whatever* is said and what is *really* said. To start, take the person and what is said at face value. Don't anticipate; don't assume with the first sentence that you know what the speaker's about to say. Avoid pre-judging and suspend judgment as you listen. You'll have plenty of time for discernment and judgment when they've finished speaking. In your response, avoid put downs or ridicule.

CHOICES

Listen below your defenses. This can be tough unless you've worked through the previous chapters. Don't assume everything said refers to you personally. Even if the other person is name-calling, be okay—that's hard, but your objective is not to strike back. Instead, as part of listening actively, voice what you hear them saying under or with the anger. Don't "return fire" to verbal abuse or name-calling.

Listening below your defenses, however, doesn't mean you submit to abuse. If the speaker is out of control, call a time out. You might say, "[name], I would like to pursue this issue with you but shouting (name-calling,) is not helpful." If the speaker does not respond positively to this request, then you might withdraw, saying that you will talk with them later. Then be sure to reopen the topic at a later time when they have cooled off or are in a better frame of mind. If the speaker is really out of control, you may need to withdraw with a calm word or saying, "Stop. You are hurting me." Vent your own upset by writing down your observations and responses and working them through before you reopen conversation.

Respond to what you hear and understand. To do this you need to use some of the techniques for talking from the next section. Your goal is to respond in a way that moves the two of you to mutual understanding. So first you want to voice what you heard and understood, asking for feedback about whether you've heard clearly or not. Be sure that you aren't pursuing a hidden agenda in your response (such as trapping the other in an inconsistency—a subtle put down). In responding, it's okay to draw from your own experience if that makes the matter under discussion clearer. Such response and clarification will usually open the way for going forward toward understanding.

Techniques for Talking

Your goals for talking are to communicate your thoughts and feelings clearly and in a way that they can best be "heard" and "understood." Talking should not be a weapon to injure the other or a shield to shut out the other. These techniques can help.

Talking in the moment—be there! This technique is the verbal partner to Listening in the Moment. When conversing with another person, place 100% of your attention on communicating. Drop what you are doing, take a deep breath, and relax. Focus on the other person, make eye contact and share what you wish to say. Avoid thinking about next steps to reach your goal in the conversation or thinking about what you have to do next. Even if you have a meeting in 15 minutes, approach the conversation directly but as if you had all the time in the world. Keep what you're saying simple. D o n ' t patronize the other person or use name calling or sarcasm.

Talking from the heart—mean it! Be transparent, be true to yourself in what you say. Open yourself to risk of communication; that means you must be sincere in attitude and choice of words. Avoid taking a superior attitude— for example, you might say "we have a problem," not "you have a problem." And remember, you can't fake sincerity. If you are really too angry to talk, it's okay to say, "I really want to talk about this, but I'm too hot right now and I don't want to take it out on you." If that's really the case, the other person will probably pick up on your sincerity. Even if they respond badly and start putting you down, be okay and withdraw.

Talking below your defenses. This technique is a partner to Listening Below Your Defenses, and it's equally hard. Your goal is to keep your perspective, that is a little distance, on the dialogue or exchange. This means always choosing your words carefully so that you are talking beneath your anger. If the other person labels, pushes buttons, or name calls, don't take the bait. Till you get some practice avoiding that bait, you may have to follow that old advice, "If you can't say something nice, Thumper, just don't say anything at all." Take a deep breath and taste those words before you speak.

In many tough conversations, you may need to discuss some hurt. When that's the case, be brief; don't go on and on about how you feel. Long-windedness about your pain will probably just make the other person defensive. Even if you are responding to something the other has said about you and you've determined that what they're saying really is about you and not themselves, try to focus on their feedback—and respond without heat to that.

CHOICES

Choosing your words carefully. If you want meaningful dialogue, then choosing words is important. To be heard and not to have what you say deflected requires taking emotionalism, not feeling, out of the words you say and the tone in which you say them. Using the baiting approach of talk radio, then, will be counterproductive. Talk radio often baits listeners just so they will "react" rather than engage in a meaningful exchange of ideas.

Using "I" Statements rather than "You" Statements. I have shared this technique previously. It's one of my favorites because it is so effective. When you are upset or bothered by some behavior that seems to be directed at you, rather than accuse the other person, you make a statement about how you are feeling. You speak with calmness and clarity of thought and emotion. You exchange "I" statements for accusatory "you" statements. You voice your issue clearly without judging or blaming—you choose your words.

For example, let's say that your spouse is late for the agreed upon departure time for the umpteenth time. Of course, while you are trying to get to your event is probably not the time to raise the issue, but you can't help stewing about it. So what do you do?

This very common complaint in relationships is also one of the hardest to address in a positive way that moves toward a solution rather than an argument. Consequently, your first step is to quit stewing, to chill, to place the incident in perspective. To take positive action you must be in a receptive, listening mode. You can't be that if you are still stewing. You also don't want to set your spouse up for a fall—that too would be counterproductive.

As you chill, mentally ask is this about me or about them? Or is it mixed? What might be the deeper issues? After reflection, at an appropriate opportunity make an "I" statement (rather than an accusatory statement). For example, your spouse may remark on how enjoyable the evening was. You might agree that you had a great time, too. Then you might say, "However, I can't help but get tensed up when for some reason we are late. I feel helpless because I don't know what to do to help us get there on time." This "I" statement sets out your difficulty and invites a response.

A number of things could happen in this response to your statement. Even though you've tried not to be judgmental, your spouse may respond as if you were placing blame. In that case, you can say, no, you just want to understand and share your problem so you can reach a joint solution. Your spouse may respond by giving a reason, for instance, "I can't get myself ready and the children set at the same time." If you aren't helping, offer to share the responsibility or to have the babysitter come earlier, for example. You might also discover you and your spouse have different views of the importance of being on time. Any and all of this data can help you work together on conflicts.

Techniques for Thinking

Communicating with a person with whom you have a relationship is not a one-time conversation, but an ongoing dialogue. Continuing to grow in relationship and in understanding means taking time to reflect on what you've heard and learned as a foundation for going forward. Taking time for reflection is particularly important when you're dealing with heated feelings. Many of the techniques you've used to help clarify your understanding of your own goals and values, feelings and facts, experiences and memories, will help in exploring your communication and relationship with another.

Journaling. Writing down your feelings and reflections soon after they happen can help you quit standing in the light. Particularly when you've had an emotional exchange (perhaps in spite of your best efforts to avoid it), jotting down your feelings can help you get distance and perspective. Put down impressions, stream of consciousness on your smart phone, tablet, or a piece of paper you keep in a pocket. Later write it up, reflecting on the various factors you see playing a role in communication or blocking it. Remember that clarity of thought usually comes when you are able to strip away the opacity of emotion, turmoil, and tension.

Problem-solving. Use your reflections (mental or journaled) to identify one or two specific blocks to communication that you'd like to work on or one or two things about yourself that you'd like to change to enhance communication. Identify one or two steps or techniques to help you start working on that goal. Plan

CHOICES

To evaluate how you did. Pull in your work from Chapter 5; use those techniques. And keep on keeping on.

The hierarchy of behavior is one more thing to keep in mind. Keep looking at the overall picture and remember that attitudes filter from top down, where behavior or action reflects off the top. Thus, behavior flows from bottom up. Those below you mimic you, you may unintentionally mimic those above you. It happens in families and in businesses. As we have discussed, these phenomena recycle in families: children mimic parents. Business also behave like families in many ways: employees mimic bosses or follow their demands out of fear and out of sheer resentment. At work, as at home, the "troops" can undermine the boss's or parents' interests. The message is clear: when it's appropriate for you to be the adult, then be one. And it's good sense to invest in everyone you influence wherever you are.

12

Life's Big Dance—Connecting as a Couple

In this chapter

- Explore how marriage relationships have a profound impact on individual well-being, including physical and psychological health.

- Examine how many stresses and joys in the life of a couple arise from individual choices each partner makes.

- Explore how to build a more committed identity as a unified "we" based on better self understanding.

- Avoid the pit-falls, stumbling blocks and blind-spots and find the techniques you need to support the unity of "we."

Our relationships are truly affairs of the heart—they have a profound impact on our well-being, including our physical and psychological health. For most adults, no relationship in life is more important than that we share with our spouse. In one aspect, at least, science confirms this importance because demographic studies have shown that married individuals tend to live longer than divorced or single persons.

When you fell in love and dreamed of establishing your own home, you may have pictured a peaceful, loving atmosphere in which both of you excelled in supporting each other and meeting each other's needs: the perfect dance of well-matched partners. Yet in reality, this relationship is usually as stressed and threatened as your individual life. In fact, many of the stresses as well as the joys arise from individual choices each person makes within the relationship. And everyone makes those choices based on their working models and self understanding, including all the inherited behaviors from their original families, modifications, and adaptive choices. So to connect fully and positively as a couple, you need to work within that relationship to use feelings as cues to facts and to use the insights gained to help you learn how to enhance, rather than destroy, your life's big dance.

What Is the Ideal Connectedness We Strive For?

By ideal, I don't mean a romantic fantasy but rather a vision of an achievable way of being and growing together as self-aware, whole persons who are equal partners in the dance of life.

Being vitally connected requires being independently dependent. Such partners will

- know "me"
- value "we"
- stay tuned to "thee"

Such partners connect, first and last, as friends—unique, vital best friends. This is connecting at a life-giving level—a level that nurtures physical and emotional health. When you connect this way as a couple, the whole is greater than the sum of the parts—the two individuals. Paradoxically, there is great freedom in connecting in such a way.

What Is the Reality We Too Often Achieve?

Broken—or in need of repair—but fixable.

You, like every one of us, aren't a finished being—not when you fell in love, not when you married, not now. That fact plays an important role in the daily dynamics of relating to a life partner and in the patterns of relating to one another you create over time.

Each partner brings to a new relationship at least three people—oneself and one's parents. Previously married people bring even more people into the relationship. All too often each partner's working model (which most people haven't thought about, much less tried to understand) grows from what was absorbed in childhood—particularly the dynamics of how one's parents related to each other. As a result, newly married partners often start by recycling behaviors that are not best for the new relationship—unaware that these deeply-rooted behaviors are inherited.

Each partner also brings his or her burdens of unresolved hurts and griefs, which so often underlie the goals, dreams, expectations and aspirations of a new relationship. History accumulates. Partners not only bring personal history to the relationship but together they also create a history, a past, and patterns as a couple and family. This history is affected not just by the relationship between husband and wife but by relationships with children, extended family, friends, and co-workers.

Working From Your Reality Toward a Shared Ideal—the Focus of This Chapter

To work toward the goal of connecting as a couple, what are we going to do in this chapter?

- Look at how many of the issues you explore for yourself in Part I play out in your relationship as a couple.

- Illustrate common dynamics with stories/experiences of real couples. Each couple is unique, but the patterns of the dance are shared.

- Review techniques for exploring, communicating, and building positive interactions that I shared in Chapter 9.

- Set goals for achieving better awareness, better management and better choices to strengthen your connection as a couple.

CHOICES

I
The Issues

Pitfalls & Perils—The Bumps on the Dance Floor

What are the elephants that keep breaking into and stomping all over your dance?

The baggage you both bring

All couples bring positive and negative working models from their families of origin as a "dowry" to their new relationship. Failing to understand your baggage and how it conflicts with your partner's baggage (and it always will) creates a big bump or block in your partnership's dance. This baggage contains not only hurts and griefs (that you probably unconsciously hoped the new relationship would heal) but it also contains personal values and goals you see as personal strengths or positives. That was true for Kimberly and Ted.

When Kimberly and Ted met at a college mixer, they were instantly attracted to one another. Ted's wicked wit—he was always ready with a snappy observation or comeback—softened by his lopsided grin charmed Kimberly. It was comfortable, for a change, to be with a guy who didn't seem to take life too seriously. Sure he was a little rough and crude at times, a little too sarcastic, maybe took jokes a little too far, but he seemed right for her. Her dad also approached almost everything as the fit object for his sarcastic wit. And except when that sarcasm was directed at her, Kimberly had enjoyed it.

Ted blossomed with Kimberly's acceptance. Even if she gently, hesitantly chided him occasionally, she gave him space and cut him some slack. She wasn't always on his case like the folks at home. As long as he could remember, Ted's parents had been immersed in their insurance business. They were always down at the office, and at dinner time they were watching the TV news and not very communicative. Even a few jokes to liven things up got put down. He assumed they were proud of him only because a friend might say, "Your dad was bragging about that ribbon you got at the science fair" or something like that. So Ted relished Kimberly's attention and acceptance; he could even put up with her occasional protests or suggestions.

You won't be surprised to learn that various problems began to spill out of their baggage in the years after Ted and Kimberly married, finished university, started their family and built Ted's business career. Kimberly grew more and more frustrated because Ted rarely followed through on promises, even when she kept reminding him and trying to help him do better. Ted was irritated by Kimberly's habits of seizing the moral high ground and holding up her "pretty rigid" code of right and wrong as superior to his. Who could live up to Miss Perfect? So he turned his sharp tongue on her, punching some holes in that self-righteousness. If she tried to come back at him, he just withdrew.

Well, she was a Christian, wasn't she? Kimberly thought: she was big enough to let the hurts go and get on with it. She felt she had done just that in their many years of marriage.

"Right!" said Ted, "If you think you are all forgiveness and light, why can you recite chapter and verse of every sin you think I've committed against you?"

"Give it a rest, Ted. You are just striking out at me to try to cover up the fact that you don't do what you say you will. You're trying to blame me for your problems."

"And you're not?"

Stalemate—once again.

It's not my problem, it's yours

In this last exchange, Kimberly and Ted have tripped over another huge bump. Placing blame on your partner is always a dead end. Playing the blame game can take many forms. In addition to direct accusation of responsibility, one popular way to blame the other is to hold yourself up as an example of the "right way to do it"—whatever *it* is. Giving unsolicited advice—even with the best intentions—can be perceived as blaming. The partner placing blame usually casts herself or himself as victim as well. Even if you've judged correctly that your partner is acting in ways that hurt you, and in that sense you are a victim, it's a mistake to take refuge in victimhood or to assume that "being wronged" places you in a superior moral or emotional position. Resting on your laurels or perceived high ground as victim is a trap.

Blame labels your partner. And remember that everyone tends to live down to labels. The response to blaming and labeling is not usually change or a positive response. Blaming, a form of attack, usually leads to denial, defensiveness, and/or withdrawal and avoidance. Defensiveness may take the form of explaining oneself, often over and over again. You may have noticed that when Kimberly scolds Ted, he tends to skirt the issue and growl, bouncing the attack and responsibility back at Kimberly. And she jabs back.

If the blame game is a constant part of your dance, as it is for Ted and Kimberly, you may discover that when either of you perceives even the slightest hint of criticism, you fall right into the typical blame responses. These patterns of blame are dead ends. Remember the only person you can change is yourself. Of course, issues need to be aired, shared and addressed, but use the techniques of the previous chapter, not to blame, but to help you move forward. Blame just keeps each partner dug in behind their armored walls.

Just who's in charge here? And whose job is it really?

As Mark moved frequently from state to state during his youth, he discovered that being a bluffer and a bully worked for him. He could soon win a place in the new school and circle of friends that not only felt safe but gave him authority. He carried this mode over into adulthood and into his career as he built a powerful public relations and advertising firm. At his agency, there was no question about who was the supreme authority. He set the standards; and he hired and fired to fit them. As old hands reminded new hires, Mark had been known to fire employees from the top V.P. to the lowliest runner just because one piece of work fell short of perfect.

Mark had married Laura, who seemed ideally matched with such an autocratic perfectionist. Growing up as one of seven in a family where the children were to be seen little and heard less (children weren't allowed to speak at the dinner table until they reached age sixteen), Laura was quiet and dutiful. Although Laura had a successful career in a commercial design firm, friends remarked that she seemed content to follow Mark's lead in everything.

When he set the rules, she was a stickler for following them and keeping order. On the surface, their marriage seemed the perfect match for two fairly extreme personalities. But the facts below the surface reveal a different reality.

Mark was so driven to success on his terms, so fueled by buried anger that it came as no surprise to his physicians when he developed multiple health issues (including a major heart attack) by his late forties. Meanwhile, Laura tended to choke back her feelings, letting them grow inside until she exploded. Then she'd vent unexpectedly. In her anger, she'd resemble a small lizard puffing itself up to ward off a much larger predator. Such tantrums often ended with crazy ultimatums: "we get rid of this stupid dog—I can't stand that dog's hair everywhere—or I go. I mean it." Her family didn't know whether to laugh at or fear these freakish outbursts. The 14-year-old son, the only child still at home, just tried to slide away. Mark was genuinely afraid (in light of his many health problems and all he'd "put her through") that one day she really would leave him.

Given their personal modes of operation and the history of their relationship, the simplest encounters often unpredictably tapped into all the buried confusions, conflicts, and hurts and escalated out of control. Consider what happened when Mark and Laura decided to "spend more time together" by having a regular "movie night out" for the two of them. They hoped it would improve things.

One day as Mark raced home, a little behind schedule, to pick Laura up for dinner for their first Friday movie date, he mentally clicked through several options, deciding as he pulled into the driveway that he'd prefer the new Al Pacino film. Bounding into the house, he saw Laura coming down stairs all ready to go. *Hey*, it occurred to him, *she must really want to go.* Then, just as he was about to say, "All ready for dinner and that Al Pacino film?" the thought flashed that maybe he ought to ask what she wanted to see. So he did, saying "I thought we'd go to the Blue Parrot for dinner, then what show do you want to see?"

Seeming pleased he'd asked, Laura responded quickly, "What about the new Harrison Ford movie?"

Surprised (and a bit irritated) at her quick response, Mark hesitated a nanosecond too long. Laura began to wilt and withdraw,

"But that's okay. You don't want to see that do you? What do you want to see?"

Mark took a deeper breath, visibly getting a grip, "No, no...we'll see what you want to see.

"But you don't want to."

"That doesn't matter," Mark began to clench his jaw. "You said you wanted to be consulted more in making our decisions, and I'm consulting you."

"But when it's clear you'd really rather do something else, it'll be easier to do what you want. . . . " As Laura's voice trailed off, Mark felt caught out in the wrong again. Soon the simple decision of what movie to see had left Mark and Laura at cross purposes and seething with irritation. The evening had become one more stumbling block rather than a positive opportunity.

Early in life, Mark had discovered that "command and demand," rather than dialogue and discussion between equals, got him what he wanted the quickest. Using that style was soon an engrained habit at work and at home. Laura had certainly grown up with an extreme example of a command-and-demand father while her mother modeled the silent stoic. Although Laura outwardly accepted these models and stuffed her feelings, she felt invisible. Over the years her suppressed anger festered just below her consciousness. Both Mark and Laura have unresolved issues about their "rights." Mark is fairly vocal about getting what he wants, and if he hurts some feelings, he believes he has a right to a little slack. Being catered to, even pampered is also his right. Laura appears to buy into that approach but deep within she resents it. She'd like to be "considered as a person" at home like she is at work, but she is not really sure about what she wants and certainly is not comfortable with expressing herself.

It's very clear to anyone observing their interactions that Mark and Laura are not working as a team. They also can't communicate clearly about what each expects of the other. Mark typically acts out a "boss and junior partner" style of decision-making, and although Laura internally resists and resents being cast as that "junior partner," she has trouble articulating her desires clearly and tends to cave into old patterns of buying peace by cutting Mark slack. Both need to practice treating the other as they would like to be treated and really communicating and listening to each other. For example, on movie night out, what if Laura had not just caved, but said, "But maybe you had a different movie in mind. Tell me what it is and then let's look at which one we'd both like to see most." With this response she's treated Mark's "consultation" as an opportunity to really discuss what they'd like to see, no matter how reluctant or insincere the subtext of Mark's question feels to her. She doesn't just cave to his wishes but allows him to enter into a more equal exchange, while both get to save face.

I'm listening, but I can't hear you

Jim and Fran have been married about 15 years, a second marriage for both. At present, Jim's recovering from heart surgery. He's always been a grump, who tends to focus on perceived catastrophes—his own or the world's. In rehab group recently, he was huffing that he felt like a victim of technology—bypass surgery and a new pacemaker were keeping him from getting back to his "old" self. As his voice and, no doubt, his blood pressure rose, Fran intervened quietly but supportively. Level headed and with good ideas, she reminded Jim gently of the possibility of using what he perceives as catastrophe as an opportunity to make some of the changes he's said he wants. To me as the facilitator and to others in the group, Fran's manner and suggestions seemed just right. But Jim wouldn't allow himself to be comforted.

As he responded to what she'd said, it was apparent that where others saw new methods and opportunities, Jim was hearing only bashing, instantly linking Fran to past hurts and to behaviors he associated with his first wife and his mother. Stubbornly clinging to the past, he was layering old grievances onto new circumstances, and treating Fran, who truly is a very different person, as if she were his first wife or had inherited in some mysterious way all her faults. In the exchanges between husband and wife, Jim was listening to what Fran said just to counter her attempts at comforting him. He belittled her suggestions, excusing himself for his behavior or choices, and making jokes at Fran's expense. She stayed calm and focused for a while, but as her frustration sharpened, so did her comments. Finally, neither was really hearing the content of what the other was saying. Jim in particular seemed to be looking only for an opening into which he could drive the last word.

I might as well be talking to the wall

This piece of baggage is the flip side of "I'm listening, but I can't hear you." Frank and Cynthia are both masters of wall-building. Frank, in particular, is a grand master of the stonewall, an interesting attribute in a man whose career is in one of the helping professions. Within their relationship, both expect to be understood through indirect communication. Rather than make clear statements, each appears to think that the other should just intuit their desires or opinions and gets miffed when understanding doesn't occur.

When Frank gets angry, a rather frequent occurrence, he shuts down. He can stay silent for days when he feels ignored, accused, misunderstood, or under-appreciated. Lots of the fights occur when Frank's mess—his piles of papers—spills out of the room they've agreed is his space to keep as cluttered as he likes, and into the living spaces they share. Frank thinks she ought to cut him "a little slack." Cynthia thinks he ought to stick to the compromise; she feels like she's keeping her side of the bargain. When, no matter how kindly, Cynthia points out that Frank's papers have begun to take over the kitchen and family room, he usually says nothing, may move a few things off the coffee table and back to "his" room (the dining room), and then simply ignores Cynthia.

Originally, Cynthia kept whacking verbally at Frank to try to break through the wall of silence, only to learn that confrontation just prolonged the deep-freeze treatment. So she adopted silence, too. Their standoffs can go on for hours or days but always continue until one or the other can find a way to resume direct verbal communication without appearing to concede victory to the other. Both partners, but particularly Frank, are behaving in code and expecting to be read. Both partners, but particularly Cynthia, feel they are talking to impervious rocks. Frank thinks that Cynthia knows what he's like, that she knew what he was like all those years before they got married, and that he gives the "mess thing" his best try and Cynthia should just understand and live with it. Cynthia's attitude is, why waste my energy and breath on trying to persuade a man who clearly has no ears and who acts so childishly.

Would it surprise you to learn that both Frank and Cynthia were the babies in their families of origin?

Setting your partner up for a fall — Baiting, button pushing, and labeling

Using coded behavior and expecting it to be read (pouting, "humpfing" around the house, slamming stuff—and many more subtle actions), then getting upset when the behavior is not read or picked up is a type of baiting. Frank and Cynthia do this a lot.

Baiting also includes the practices of button pushing and labeling that I discussed in Chapter 4. When you have a close relationship such as that between spouses, it's very easy for one partner to bait the other. We often do so by pushing buttons of sensitivity or labeling and thus triggering the baited partner's reactivity. Gottcha—you've caught them in your trap or lured them off the cliff.

Baiting is one of the most common ways that couples fight, but it's not fighting fair because it's deliberately taking advantage of a partner's weakness. These tactics achieve the opposite results of the desirable end which is to "air and repair" grievances. Sometimes after we have the other person flopping on the hook, we give it an extra yank by holding our own behavior related to the grievance up as the model. If we could only see our inner "grin" when the other grabs that dangling bait-disguised hook, we might be ashamed of ourselves and quicker to work on the goal of really listening, identifying the problem (is this about me or about them?), letting go any baggage that gets in the way, and really trying to respond to the grievance.

Out-of-bounds behavior

In the extreme, some of these behaviors that I've been describing can be abusive verbally, emotionally, or physically. Abuse occurs when you violate personal space and appropriate boundaries—not just the other person's defined boundaries but the appropriate limits to your own behavior. Out-of-bounds behavior is doing unto the other what you would not want done to you.

CHOICES

Although physical injury may come most quickly to mind at the mention of "abuse," I find that many couples who would never physically strike one another, often think nothing of verbally and emotionally abusing each other. To give an example of such emotional abuse, one partner might share something special which the other then reveals inappropriately to others. In revealing the confidence, the abuser often presents it to the audience as something to ridicule. The tone can be light and the speaker deprecating while the actual words patronize, stab or cut the partner or child who's being made fun of.

When tempted to make a joke at your partner's expense, ask yourself, if I were the "butt" would this be funny or hurtful, amusing or insulting? If you find that such out-of-bounds behavior is a frequent or uncontrollable part of the way you relate to others or you see nothing wrong with it, seeking appropriate professional counseling to help you overcome these problems would be a wise and courageous choice.

II

What's Our Real Story?
Finding the Facts Behind Our Feelings and Behaviors as a Couple

What was your goal in marriage or becoming a couple? Were you trying to recreate your family of origin or create a new bonded relationship built on shared values and mutual respect for individuality and differences? Which have you done? To what degree have you mixed these approaches together? Or pulled in other factors? Where would you like to go as a couple? How would you like to connect?

To find the answers to these questions, you will need to look for the facts behind your feelings and behaviors—your dance—as a couple. If you can share and communicate about these matters openly, that's a big head start. And then as a couple, you can certainly use some of the exercises that I presented in Chapters 5 and 6.

But more often, partners are at different places in the journey of understanding. So even as a partner you must start by looking at yourself and at the facts behind your feelings and behaviors in the relationship. You can observe your partner, you can listen carefully to what she or he says, but you can't speak for your partner and you can't change your partner. Remember your sphere of influence—you can only change yourself. But all your actions and interactions can enhance and help build your relationship or tear it down. Your expectations, words, and behaviors can bait your partner or set him or her up positively. You won't know how until you dive down and understand what's going on and where it comes from.

III

Freeing Yourselves as a Couple to Connect and Grow

Connecting as a couple is not easy, but the effort is worth it. In the life of every couple there are times when it's easier to say, "yes, we need to do something different" or to admit that something is broken and needs fixing. Those are moments when our hearts are softened. These moments are the same for couples as they are for individuals. They include times of fresh starts or new beginnings such as getting married, establishing a new family, the birth of the first child and other children, for example. Other times spring from traumatic, stressful occurrences to one or both partners such as the diagnosis of a significant health problem such as heart disease, cancer or debilitating illness, the illness or death of a loved one, the loss of a job or work related failure, relocating, retiring and so forth.

In the next few sections, I outline very briefly some of the questions and techniques that you can use to go forward together.

What do you need to go forward as a couple?

It would be great if every man and woman as they begin to think about making a commitment to a life together would work seriously *as a couple* on planning for a supportive and empowering relationship. All too often, however, the rosy glow of romance clouds our vision. Many couples these days may be setting up prenuptial agreements about finances (and that's not necessarily bad), but they'd probably be much better off if they worked on some prenuptial skills for supporting and enhancing their committed relationship. Of course, it's never too late to start working on this goal. What does it take?

- An overview of expectations and personal history, opinions, and values from both people.
- Education for new insights.
- Common language—define and redefine terms; learn how to stay talking.
- Planning for how to interact, to go forward. It's a great idea to set an actual time to do this regularly—at an anniversary (not on the day), or a weekend off together.
- Planning for negative days, backsliding, pitfalls. You can't escape some conflict; you have to handle it positively using "I" statements and other techniques.

Where's your focus? What's important?

What you value determines your focus. Remember you are seeking clarity. Remember the important triad of Me, We, Thee. Your first commitment is to being a couple—a We.

As a couple, you share responsibility and leadership— enjoy team play— enhance the DANCE. Sharing is not anarchy—too often we think of "leadership" in hierarchical or military terms (i.e. officers lead soldiers, the head chef commands the cooks). In sharing leadership, good teams do define roles and responsibilities, but they define them together and they learn how to hand off or share responsibility as necessary

What will it take to achieve your goals as a couple?

First, you need to be committed to good communication. You need to define mutual goals—though you may need to work through some of the personal tasks below (and in previous sections) to be able to do that. You also need to understand that achieving your desired connection as a couple not only nurtures the emotional safe haven you want your home to be but also nurtures your and your partner's physical well-being.

When two people come together they have an ideal image. To achieve that ideal (or even something close to it) you need to release and be released from your baggage. To draw from a biblical image, you need to go to a new land of Canaan, where there's milk and honey on the other side but a different kind of milk and honey from the positives of childhood. Each person has to let go the bad, use the positives (not inflict them on your partner), and together create new definitions for the "We." Then together you need to re-evaluate these definitions on a regular basis.

Understanding yourself

This is the lesson of Part I of this chapter—you must first discover and understand your own realities and ideals, positive and negative, if you wish to connect most fully and successfully with the one you love.

Affirm the "We": Recognize your partner as your equal— the dance takes two

When two people behave as a couple, their interactions are not about control, power, or authority, but about meeting the needs and fulfilling the desires of the couple and each individual. Fulfilling your contribution to being a couple also means always taking responsibility to test your personal needs and desires to make sure that they are realistic and fair to the relationship as well as yourself. Being a "we" is about a connection with an equal distribution of power and resources that empowers each partner—man or woman—with clear but interchangeable responsibilities. There is more flexibility in this model, because it allows, even encourages,

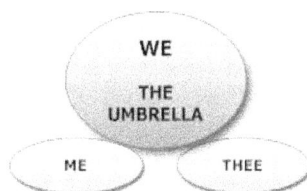

.

WE

THE
UMBRELLA

ME   THEE

compromise and change as necessary. The "WE" is essentially the umbrella under which the couple is bonded, their connectedness. It serves as the unit to which each member responds.

I, therefore, "do" and "be" for the relationship, the "WE," which includes my spouse, not just for me or my spouse. After all, if I continue to "do" just for my spouse, I eventually may harbor resentment, for there is usually a silent assumption that a return is expected (and deserved). It's difficult to maintain the effort unless we uncover the hidden unrealistic expectations.

The task for each partner in a couple is to commit himself or herself to working together.

- Work together back-to-back to protect your relationship from outside harm, to deal with issues, fears, and threats.
- Work together face-to-face to communicate clearly, to listen effectively to implement your agreed-upon real world strategy with the plans that you've put in place.

First and foremost, you must remember and remind yourself and each other that you are first and last *friends*; you have a deep friendship, respect and commitment that hold you together as a "we" whatever events or circumstances may come your way.

Stay tuned to "Thee"

We no longer use "thee" in everyday English. But grammatically, it's the familiar "you"—the term used for those you know best (similar to the French *tu* or German *du*). That's why I chose the word to signify the one you hold dearest.

Ches and Maria were married over fifty years before her death. It was clear to all who knew them that these folks had stayed best friends for all those years, through the good times and the bad times (and there'd been some doozies healthwise and economically). But they clearly brought joy to themselves, to their family, and to friends spread all over the country. What was their secret, their niece asked one day. "Well," Ches replied, "I can't speak for Maria, but I've tried to court her every day of my life." Knowing how Maria had enthusiastically joined Ches in all his adventures including those others might have said were impossible "at your age" or "without more money in the bank" suggested that Maria did the same. Never forget that your partner is the beloved—even when you are mad at them.

Claim opportunities to start over

But let's say that your marriage, like most folks', has not been one long, care-free courtship. Our experiences don't match the ideal of our newly-wed dreams. When we enter a new relationship, there's the unspoken hope that each partner will keep their vows warm and close to their heart and express them (cherish the other) through every action. The rosy images of romance we're fed daily turn out to be so much balderdash. We soon learn that marriage is hard work.

No couple plans to turn their new relationship into a reflection of the original ones from which they came. No one plans to recreate the dance they grew up with and are thus familiar with deep inside. Even if you think you've run in the opposite direction from the negative aspects of the relationship you grew up in, when the stresses of building a day-in day-out relationship arise, you will fall right into those patterns unless you have examined your roots for yourself (hopefully your spouse will do his/hers) and together discuss and choose what will affirm and work best for your "WE" not somebody else's "WE."

The best wedding gift that parents can give children is permission and encouragement to make their relationship new. Every father, every mother, ought to take their son or daughter aside and say, "We love you. We built our marriage our way—we've made some great choices and some awful choices. You and your spouse-to-be are not us. You are you. Wipe the slate clean. We want you *together* to build *your* model for marriage. You have our absolute permission to build it new. Our expectation is not that you will carry on any kind of tradition but that you place your whole heart and allegiance in your new relationship. When you do that and build it strongly, we will honor it and have confidence that the bonds of the whole extended families will be strengthened."

Unfortunately, too few parents are clear-sighted and secure enough about their own relationships and struggles to do this. Too few couples can see beyond the glow of first connections or are self-aware or secure enough to get down in the trenches and hash out an understanding of shared beliefs, values, goals, fears, and free-doms.

Fortunately, it's never too late to start over. It's healthy to start over. It may be most productive if both you and your partner agree that as a couple you need a fresh start. But even if it's just you, you can take many steps to help your partner and your relationship grow positively. For some couples, one partner or the other simply can't or won't choose to change. Making it new sometimes in the end may involve splitting up for self-preservation. You ultimately only have control and responsibility for yourself (remember your cylinder of influence) and staying in an abusive relationship is not healthy. But thankfully, most couples can embrace more hope and make more healthy changes. Here—as a couple or for yourself—are some of the important goals and techniques in starting over.

Let go the negative and unhelpful

What are some of the most important things to let go?
- The desire to change or remake the other—you can't do it
- The desire to CONTROL the other
- The burdens of the past—explore them, understand their power, let the bad baggage go
- Hanging on to hurts—don't bury hurts but express them appropriately before they fester; communicate individual problems when you recognize them, don't let them smolder
- The urge to explain, explain, explain
- Having to have the last word
- Labeling the other—a way of excusing self, hanging on to hurts, belittling the other

Be present in the moment for the other

You can choose to be up front and transparent, to shed your armor (even if that's scary) and risk vulnerability. The positives of "getting naked" work at psychological and emotional levels as they do on the physical level.

What will it take for you to reveal yourself? How can you help your partner do the same?
- Speak clearly from facts

- Use clear communication techniques such as "I statements"
- Observe, listen and ask questions based on what will move you both ahead

Learn to say "I'm sorry" and follow-up with action that proves it

If you've reached outside of your cylinder of influence or boundaries and "slugged" your partner inside their cylinder, then you must first act to make your partner feel better. Typically, we say, "I'm sorry." But words alone are not enough—you must really acknowledge and take responsibility for your actions. Your words will ring hollow, or even become a nagging irritant, unless you take active steps to change the behavior that you are sorry about. The promise and the steps you take don't need to be huge; the first step just needs to be one simple thing that addresses the immediate complaint: For example, "Yes, I will call next time I'm going to be late" or "I won't tell that story on you again" or "I will not be late for our next date (and if I'm held up at work unavoidably I will take time to call)."

But what if you're not sure that you really have done any-thing wrong? Remember always to ask yourself in moments of conflict or complaint, *is this about me or about them*? If it is really your partner's issue, then you need to keep working on letting go your own irritation. Try to listen to the real message under your partner's words and actions. Use non-threatening "I" statements to clarify or to reflect what you hear and what you feel. Stay calm. Be okay and transparent in the moment. If it's truly about them, don't say "I'm sorry" just to deflect being involved in the moment—that will only complicate matters. You may, of course, need to withdraw if the other is too heated; you might say something such as, "I want to listen and talk about this, but only when you've cooled down." Valuing the "we" and the "thee" means committing yourself to the relationship.

Listen to feedback from your partner

If both of you are calm (or after a cool down period), really listen to what your partner is saying. Listen beneath your defenses.

CHOICES

This means first asking yourself, is this about me or about them? If it's about them, listen and watch carefully. What's your perception? What do you see beneath the anger? Whatever's fueling the anger is real—even if you don't feel that the other's anger is justified. Just because your partner pops off about something and part of what is said points at you, making you squirm with guilt and defensiveness, you don't have to react. Reflect and respond as appropriate. Stay calm and wait. Listening doesn't mean being a doormat, even when it means being okay and being transparent. After a moment, try again.

If your partner's concern or problem really is about you, listen and respond willingly. What in your partner's statement is valid? What is not? If you are okay and don't get defensive no matter what the issue or your perception of the validity of your partner's perception or accusation, you'll be surprised at how your being okay and calm can usually defuse the tension and heat.

If the other is so angry that he or she is beyond hearing or is verbally abusive, it's okay to withdraw, but not to run away. Say simply and calmly, "I want to talk about this with you but not when you are so angry. I can't really listen or hear you properly when your words make me feel ____ (fill in the blank accurately, for instance, "hurt," "intimidated," "uncomfortable," "bewildered," or "frightened"). Then at the earliest convenient moment when the other is cool, initiate the conversation.

Working together is give-and-take—it's dancing

Living and growing in a healthy, life-sustaining relationship is like dancing—like moving together through space and time, stepping and feeling together, creating a pattern that's unique to who you both are. There's mutual give-and-take. There's a recognition of strengths and shifting leadership. There's sensitivity to what's going on with the partner.

The dance my wife and I have created through the years seems best described as a "rolling" process. One action gets us from here to there and we each can depend on it. We each have on call our compensations, our determinations to be there for the other, our defenses to ward off the harder struggles—a commitment to continuously improve lines of communication and understanding, and we have our unifying ideals and values, some of the tethers that bind us independently together.

There are malignant ingredients to avoid such as (a) busyness or indifference (b) multi-tasking – that too can be multi-taxing (c) pre-occupations, (d) over-attentiveness to certain details at the wrong time, (e) unrelenting teasing - too testy, (f) too much distancing – nearly to the point of uncaring or (g) too close to the issues or the other's business – overly enmeshed. The balance of what we each do for the other, what we expect to gain for ourselves and between what we say and do and what's in our hearts and comes out our mouths, these are all issues that can decide how each of us chooses to treat or react to the other. If each of us is not grounded in the unceasing, mostly selfless commitment to the relationship, to the "We," then we each become less than the "Me" we want to be. The "we" of the relationship is more important to each of us than our individual prominence. Yet we know that unless we take care of "me" and continually work on "me"—the only choices totally in one's command—we can't bring our best selves to the "we." So it's a rolling process—by committing to "we" I work to be the "me" I desire and choose; by becoming a better "me" attentive to "thee" and committed to "we" together we enjoy and heighten the sustaining, joyful dance.

Decide upon and practice family principles

As part of connecting as a couple and as you shape your family, you may find it very helpful to articulate and actually write down values or principles. Although they are open to growth and change, such family principles can become a touchstone or foundation to keep you grounded as a couple.

Here are some that form the bedrock for my wife and me.

I. We follow the golden rule—do unto others as you would have them do unto you.
II. We uphold the relationship between the parents as of primary importance to the well-being of the whole family and the children as individuals.
III. We want to help our children to bear responsibility in the family.
IV. We maintain that we're rich with blessings.
V. Our family remains steeped in positive traditions.

VI. We give respect and consideration to one another at all times.

VII.   We eat meals and take vacations together.

VIII.   We are there for each other.

Practice, practice, practice—some rules for the dance

The following list can remind you of techniques to practice so that connecting as a couple is richly rewarding.

- No advice
- No blaming
- No guilt
- No judging
- No back-pedaling
- No being defensive
- No explaining without being asked
- Be direct
- Be bold
- But think before talking
- Say what you want
- Use your words
- Choose your words
- Put reservations on the table without anger
- Be transparent
- Stay on point
- Avoid past baggage
- Don't dangle the bait
- Don't take the bait
- Respect personal boundaries
- Avoid reacting
- Focus on your issues, not your partner's
- Listen, listen, listen
- Be "in the moment"
- Appreciate lessons learned from your history
- Avoid over-processing the negative or the positive
- Avoid unrealistic expectations
- Avoid over-anticipating
- Appreciate that silence is enriching
- Back up words with behavior

The rewards of connecting as a couple

The best relationships are always works in progress. Growing together, working through issues from where you are now to where you want to go or even to where you feel more comfortable, enriched and happy in your relationship can take time. But it's rewarding to realize you're no longer practicing this dance step or that, but you and your partner are actually dancing—free-floating and light-on-your-feet—simply doing it! Such a distinct move may, in fact, be the ultimate strategy from mental vision to reality. To escape from the ever-attentiveness and burdensome practice-mode—to successfully disengage and distance ourselves from the baggage, our habits from out of the past—and to live in real-time, in-the-moment, free to negotiate the given journey with our beloved is the true, immediate gift of life. The ongoing and ultimate gifts of focusing upon strengthening the relationships with those we love are clarity in communication, clarity of emotions, clarity of choices, and—no small boon—better health.

When you have reached this step of really "dancing" together, you are able to continue to build a more fulfilling connection with each other. Such potential for living up to your stars as a couple is a gift, for you're able to put hope, practice, and theory into real life. Individually each of you can complete the journey begun early in life. Because you both have worked on yourselves and finished the uncompleted training laid down in your early childhoods and dealt with the upwelling sources of conflict, you both now have a better chance for growth and maturity in your new relationship. The vows you spoke at your wedding become a living, daily spring of hope and fulfillment and joy.

13
Nurturing Your Children for Healthy, Independent Lives

In this chapter

All parents want the best for their children. The concepts in this book offer parents helpful insights into how to nurture healthful behaviors, emotions and values in children. These approaches respect the individuality of the child and provide new ways of perceiving and influencing family dynamics. This chapter discusses the importance of visualizing the qualities of positive parenting and oneself as that ideal parent. The discussion also covers some parenting pitfalls and how to recognize and change such behaviors in yourself. Other topics include:

- The importance of expressing love to a child and ways to give that TLC
- How to positively set limits vs. meting out punishment the power of positive affirmation
- Issues of the quality and quantity of interactions with our children
- Dangers and solutions for when children get caught up into adult conflict
- Tips for physically and emotionally nurturing a healthy child at each stage of development from infancy through adolescence
- Tips for restoration. What you can do to "undo the past" if you need to.

Jake and Joanne were reminiscing with their grown daughter, Jane, about an extended cross-country family trip that they had taken twenty years earlier when Jane was a young teen. Remembering the fun they'd had, the parents were preparing Jane a scrapbook of rediscovered momentos. Jake and Joanne recalled all the historic sites and interesting places they'd visited and how hard they had worked planning the trip to be fun and educational—really working together to identify places to visit and plan a route that would be meaningful to Jane. Now twenty years later, they wondered if Jane had indeed found seeing all the sights and historic areas associated with persons important in government, science and education as educational and as enjoyable as they had hoped.

Of course, the trip stood out as very special, Jane said, but not so much for the reasons they'd identified. Certainly, she appreciated all the places, but she had most enjoyed being with them and seeing them enjoy the planning and travel together. Jane said her feeling about her parents' relationship at that time was that they did a lot of bickering and picking at each other. That had made her feel vaguely unhappy and probably a bit insecure, even guilty, as her parents sniped at each other and traded sarcastic witticisms over the breakfast and dinner tables or in the car on trips.

But as they planned this trip, she'd seen them every evening really working as a team, getting brochures, pouring over books from the library and maps, plotting out the route and using travel guides to find the best accommodations at the right price. They had worked out the trip details so well, that everything was going flawlessly. Then, mid-trip something went awry, some major glitch—she couldn't remember what—but what she did remember was that sitting in the back seat, she tensed waiting for the inevitable accusations about whose responsibility the problem was and the escalating fight. But the sniping never started. Instead, her parents solved the difficulty with the same wit and give-and-take that they'd used as they worked together planning the trip. Jane felt like her parents were interacting in new ways. That made her feel good. Before then she'd sometimes wondered if her parents were going to stay together. After the way they handled this big, unexpected problem, she felt completely different. She floated through the rest of the trip just enjoying being with them.

Jane's memory of the trip flabbergasted Jake and Joanne—her perceptions of that long-ago trip were so different from theirs. But the more they thought about it, the more they understood where she was coming from. In the months that they focused on planning the trip, they now could see that they had unconsciously been reinforcing the connections and ways of relating they had enjoyed when they courted, and the planning helped them find new ways to stay connected in the midst of more hectic work and family lives. As they planned, they were focused on a goal that they both wanted, and their primary objective was making the trip really meaningful for their daughter, not putting their own desires, tastes or whims first. In doing this, they had evolved and reinforced new patterns that strengthened their marriage then and in the future. In fact, Jane said, the way they continued to grow in communicating had become an important model for her own successful marriage.

And while she was astounding her parents, Jane thought she'd share another important lesson that she'd learned from them. This lesson had to do with being successful and competent and winning by acting from a position of self confidence, by including everyone in the game, by working together as a team and respecting the opponent. If it was a game with winning as an objective, playing one's best, rather than beating the opponent by any tactic was the goal.

She remembered that at beach vacations shared with aunts, uncles and cousins, her parents had been teaching the young children to play chess, a complex and difficult game. At first the adults always set up the chess board and invited the children to "play." These game were set so the children lost as few players as possible as they made a few simple moves. One evening, the adults were out for dinner. While the babysitting teenagers watched TV, the young ones (Jane included) wanted to play. So they got out the board and put out the pieces, arguing about the proper position of each piece and rearranging until the board met their collective satisfaction. When Jake and Joanne returned, they noted the incorrect placements and showed the "gang" all the correct positions and reminded them how to make the first moves. The children were so excited to be able to begin without the adults, that they played even more. They also enjoyed learning to negotiate and interacting with each other in the simple process. The adults in playing with the children often gave back lost pieces so that the kids could try again and learn. The fun was in playing and learning, not in winning. Everything was taken lightly. Without realizing they were studying, the children gradually learned more about the game, including how to strategize, how sometimes to "win" by losing, how to think ahead about reaching your goal, and how to observe the person you were playing with to anticipate his or her moves.

Both the chess and later the big trip, Jane said, helped her learn to look at issues from a relational basis. She learned the value of planning so that you had a "road map" that was right, not just for reaching the goals, but for doing it with the people who were on the trip or playing the game (or later, working on a business project). This structure provided her with the tools to step back to review who and what was important, to maintain her distance from the immediate by keeping her mind's eye on the overall plan, to carry out the plan and to make adjustments to that plan as she got feedback. These skills, she told her parents, were something that had served her well in her relationships with her husband, in her work, with her own children. And she pointed out, these skills she had learned primarily by observing and living them with her parents. The most powerful teaching they did was modeling by their own behaviors.

Jane's memories of lessons learned from her parents can serve as a touchstone for this chapter. Parents are our first teachers, and we usually learn from them more what we experience and observe, than what they overtly "teach." Ideally, what we teach intentionally as parents and what we convey by our own behaviors will be consistent. Each of us has gifts and burdens from the past. The bulk of this book has shared ideas and techniques to help individuals affirm health-giving behaviors and quit recycling negative ideas, values and behaviors that they have inherited. This chapter shares briefly some of the ideas and strategies you may find useful in helping your children develop values and behaviors that support their individuality, happiness and health. (I might also add that it's important to remember that it's never too late for parents to influence their children in these ways.)

A different parental scenario

"Do this!"

"Why?"

CHOICES

"Just do it!!"

"Well?!"

"Just do it!!!"

"Yes sir!!"

Dad never did say "thank you," "good job," or anything! If I were to ask him, "Why don't you explain? Why don't you praise your kids?" his response would be, "That's just the way I am." We are all the way we are. We say, " I am the way I am!"

This expression is often spoken firmly, indicating we stubbornly choose to reject change, preferring to stay the same, whatever the consequences. But in actuality, we're the way we are because of specific reasons that we've absorbed or adopted from our parents and mentors as well as from molding circumstances, events and peers.

When we become parents, we help shape our children's ways of relating to others and the world around them. What parents do you think the dad in the little scenario above is fostering? But put yourself in the child's shoes for a moment. As an adult looking back, what would have been helpful to you? Would you have wanted to understand the "whys" behind your parents' actions? Did you want your parents to understand your issues, to take time to talk to you and understand your feelings? To look at the issues from your point of view? You bet you did.

The dad in this scene who says, "just do it" is probably following a pattern he experienced as a child. Perhaps he hasn't even thought about the effectiveness of the technique. When parents move from issuing imperatives—just do it; don't do that—and start teaching from their experiences and modeling appropriate relating and problem solving, they can open up whole new opportunities to guide their children and foster healthy patterns of coping with emotions and building relationships that foster long-term health.

Setting Your Children Up for Health Starts with Looking at Your Own Issues

Whether you've only thought about it briefly or worked through the exercises in Chapters 4, 5 and 6, you can see your parents' influence in yourself. You've also hopefully come to understand the likelihood that you will transfer all the outdated behaviors (right along with positive) to your children unless you take steps to do it differently. So the first step in setting up your children for healthy growth is to deal constructively with your own issues. This outcome is one of the rewards of doing all that hard work I've outlined. Dealing with your own issues doesn't mean, by the way, always bringing them up as an example to your children (any more than to your spouse). So even if you had to "walk fifty miles in the snow and sleet without any boots" to get to school or you had to make "As" or your pop whipped your backside, don't try to use such trials as motivators for your children. Just because you had to suffer through certain painful family-inherited rites of passage doesn't mean that you have to pass on negative experiences. (Passing down such harmful negative behaviors may be the real meaning of that Biblical insight that the "sins of fathers" are visited on the children.) This form of "passing it on" is selfish and vengeful. Making your children suffer what you suffered will not get even with your parents or toughen up your children. Instead, your goal is to let go the hurts and build positive values and behaviors that set you and your children ahead.

The important foundation—being united as parents

It can also be an important plus for your children, if as parents you redefine and remake your own relationship as a couple—if you truly share hearts, if you really examine and let go the past. One of the most important requirements for positive parenting (after understanding yourself) is to be united as parents. This is true even if parents are divorced or separated. Doing the work outlined in Chapters 10, 11, and 12 is a prerequisite for positive parenting. As a couple starting a family, remember that you are starting a NEW creation—in many physical, psychological and spiritual senses. So you need to give this work the same attention and planning that you would if you were starting a new business. But in reality, most folks probably give starting a family less evaluative thought and reflection than they do to buying a new car or purchasing a house—many pay more attention to the wedding service than the actual joining in new relationship and forming a new family. Some expectant first-time parents may spend more time fixing up the baby's room than getting ready to be parents. Yet this is a great time to share your ideas of what parenting means to you, to share your golden moments in childhood and think about the kind of golden moments you'd like to enable your child to have. It's the time to think about the parenting values and techniques you share (and those you don't) and to harmonize your different approaches—to create your shared vision. In all this planning, of course, you never forget that your child will be a separate individual, not a conduit for expressing your dreams.

Basic Strategies and Principles for Parents

From the moment a baby enters the world, he or she begins to build the body and coping mechanisms that will enable them to deal with the world and its stresses. So as smart parents, you probably ought to begin envisioning and planning for the health and happiness of the child from the moment you decide to become parents. Certainly from the time you learn that he or she is on the way. Remember that behaviorally the baby will be an empty sponge as hungry to absorb experience as to take in food. Assume that as parents you will be the ones to teach the child everything. Just as you feed the baby and take care of all its bodily functions and needs, you'll also be caring for its feeling, learning self. Every moment the baby is absorbing, mimicking and processing experiences and making those experiences personal and individual. The baby will not only learn responses from those experiences but will use those behaviors to gain the attention and approval of his or her teachers—you—and to relate to others in his or her world.

One daunting fact about babies as learners is that they are non-selective learners. We joke about this truth, using familiar sayings such as "monkey see, monkey do" or "little pitchers have big ears." But the hard facts are that children take in everything, not just the specific behavior or value you wish to impart, and that they learn more from what teachers do than from what they say. This is particularly true for infants and very young children. They may focus more on the way you teach them, for example, and how you say something, than on the actual content of what you are trying to convey. That's why, for instance, if your mouth is saying "well done" to a child, but your tone is distant and your attention distracted, the child will pick up on your lack of sincere reinforcement and approval every time.

As a result, it's important to think intentionally about your own issues and how they affect your parenting as soon as possible. It's important always to remember that your purpose as a parent is to teach your children positive behaviors that help them live secure in who they are, that help them live in the moment and not cling to hurts and fears, and that help them learn to "let go" in appropriate ways for each stage of development. Your purpose is also to break any negative patterns and not to teach your children the negative emotional reactions that you may have learned growing up and that you are now trying to let go. Accomplishing these goals is hard if you are blind to some of those negative behaviors and that's why working through your own issues related to these behaviors is important.

But also remember that it's never too late to change yourself and your relationships—in that sense parenting your children, just like loving them, never ends. In fact, when you keep those pathways of communicating and giving to each other open, it's amazing that as children grow into adults and become parents we as parents have much to learn from them, too. This is particularly true when we have helped teach them to be their whole, independent, grounded selves.

Observing important boundaries as parents

The most important boundary that parents must recognize and, yes, celebrate is that each child is a simple, separate person of worth. Your child is not you. You can not live through your child or realize *your* dreams through your child. Instead, your job as parent, like mine, is to help each child live up to his or her stars not down to any labels that the child may have learned from you. We can view children as lots of trouble, as annoyances, or as interfering factors in our lives, or we can find ourselves impatient with their behaviors (even those behaviors that child development specialists assure us are typical of growing children). Even if we never actually verbalize these attitudes, our nonverbal behaviors and attitudes will inevitably communicate our true feelings. Such feelings and behaviors communicate rejection. And we should examine them and think of them as out-of-bounds in our parenting. We need to internalize the understanding that parenting is about our children, about them—not about us.

Positively, if we desire the best for our children, we can envision them as the children and young adults we want them to become. Then we will strive to speak to them, treat them, and interact with them in optimal ways that respect boundaries and help them learn to respect themselves and appropriate boundaries.

At every level of your child's development, you need to keep in mind that you are developing in parenting, too. As parents we need to continue to grow right along with our children. That means that certain expressions of boundaries and techniques we use to relate to our children will also change and grow as appropriate to their ages and to their individual personalities.

Understand you will make mistakes—and that's okay

Our lives are messy by nature; we are always learning and growing. And that means we'll make mistakes. When it comes to parenting and family relationships, for example, all those old "ropes" of reactivity still dangle before us even when we've rejected them. When a child is behaving in ways that trigger those old patterns, it's hard not to grab and yank the end of that rope that the child is throwing in front of you. When you catch yourself, for instance, constantly butting heads with a child or being critical, it's important to first ask what the situation says about you. What can you do differently to help the child achieve the behaviors and insights you are trying to instill? Are you affirming and praising as well as criticizing? What will you do differently? Course correction is always possible, particularly when we get out of our own way. So remember to re-evaluate and make changes regularly.

Issues of appropriate discipline, boundaries and punishment

Affirming your child doesn't mean that you don't set and teach appropriate boundaries. Teaching trust, responsibility and respect,

220

values that build character and health, depend on your child learning appropriate boundaries. Again, teaching appropriate boundaries proves most effective when you model those boundaries yourself and when you set boundaries for children that are clear but that respect and treat them as individuals. Certainly, children must be corrected and punished but not in ways that label them and belittle them.

One important tool is listening to your children—including "listening" to what their nonverbal behavior is telling you. If you wish your children to listen to you, then you must listen to them and respond appropriately to what you hear. When you listen and respond appropriately to what the child is thinking and feeling, then it is much easier to help the child learn boundaries and learn to reshape or correct behaviors as necessary. And in helping a child make course corrections, part of appropriate boundaries for a parent is keeping an appropriate distance from the child (not entangling our issues with the child's) and continually visualizing the positive person you want the child to be, helping them live up to their stars, not down to labels.

Some Thoughts on Parenting Boys

Earlier, I've talked about how we tend to encourage "wildness" in boys as an expected part of masculine behavior and personality. Of course, boys need exposure to the gift of wildness, but they also need equal exposure to the gift of feelings. They need to be taught to be good at communicating, listening, and connecting, to know how to sit still and be okay with rest and quiet, and to feel good about a job well done and to be able to receive both thanks and compliments. In other words, they need balance and the whole range of personal skills we've been considering in this book.

If you are a father, you have a particularly important role in helping your sons learn this balance. As dads, we enjoy teaching all the "boy skills" to our sons and other young men. But we must also teach the skills of tenderness and nurturing. To do this, let me say again, we've got to start with looking at ourselves and the behaviors we model. All too often I see men who may say to their sons, for instance, that they must respect their mothers and other women just as they would their fathers and business associates, but those words carry too little weight because how these dads treat their wives and other women contradicts their words. If we as men and husbands don't model good relationships, good communications and being okay with making mistakes and trying again to our sons and other young men with whom we work, we individually in our families (and in our society as a whole) will never stop recycling some very negative behaviors.

In some families, mothers tend to spoil their sons and cut them slack in ways they don't do for their daughters. Our cultural mores tend to reinforce this tendency. It's important for mothers and fathers to set expectations for sons that encourage them to be tender and to take responsibility for relationships and for carrying their responsibilities in the family.

Some Thoughts on Parenting Girls

What I've said about boys is also important for girls, but in many ways we need to flip the coin. With girls, parents typically (mirroring our culture in general) tend to foster in girls their skills in listening, caring, communicating and connecting—the nurturing skills. And we expect girls to be in touch with their feelings. That's great. But girls also need to experience the healthy gift of "wildness," just as we need to foster the nurturing and connecting skills in boys. Skills learned from wild activities can help girls learn more about the range of their capacities and possibilities, can help them stretch themselves to learn their limits, to open up their expectations, and to strive to achieve their full potential. Again, as for boys, balance is important. And modeling good relationships by united parents is as important for girls as for boys. Both parents need to be as available to girls as to boys.

Launching Your Children into Independent Adulthood

When do you start taking steps to "cut the apron strings," to launch your children into adulthood? If you thought, when they're teenagers, you're too late. Establishing your children as healthy, happy, successful adults starts from the moment they're born. With that thought in mind, however, remember that each step builds on the one before it. When you as parents model a sharing, mutual partnership and when you create positive family stories through the opportunities you share as a family, you are helping your children create the values they need for the future. Family stories can grow out of mundane events and special events—family supper or Thanksgiving feasts, a trip to the beach or a special birthday celebration. Each day and each encounter offers a new opportunity, one you may not even know the kids are taking in. Remember what Jane got out of that trip her mother and father planned so carefully? The important thing is to be in the moment and to be tuned in to those you care about.

Some Thoughts on Grandparenting

Grandparenting offers chances to break the recycling of negative patterns within the family. Connecting with grandchildren is not only positive in itself but it offers a great chance to connect in new, positive ways with your children. With grandchildren, you can maintain distance on the absolute responsibility of parenting and spoil a little. Because you aren't forced to be the rule makers and keepers, you can take a step back and see yourself and family patterns more clearly and *respond* to them, rather than *react* to them. You can emphasize the essence of supportive relationships. Grandparenting is a plus, a time for focusing on the gifts, joys and acceptance of your grandchildren and then your children.

As grandparents, we can more easily relate to our children as adults, exhibiting friendships as adults. Because we've distanced ourselves a step, we can be more accepting of ourselves, our faults and shortcomings and more accepting of our children. In our grandparent role, it can be easier to put the insights we've learned about ourselves and relationships into action. As we let our experiences teach us that we can only change ourselves and not others, we can then realize that small changes in ourselves can have positive effects on those we wish to influence. Hopefully, by the time we're grandparents we've learned when to keep our mouths shut and just butt out. With grandchildren, our hearts are softened. Often we find it easier to make the small sacrifices in letting go ourselves and changing for others' gain. To lose ourselves in this way is really, in my experience, to find ourselves more richly and truly.

CHOICES

A Final Thought

Parenting is the most important job you'll ever have in your life—and the hardest. It's also the most rewarding. As you think about enhancing your loving relationships with your children, remember these two things: 1) Every day is a new day with the possibility of new beginnings and new opportunities to show your children your love, support and guidance. 2) It's never too late to begin—and the first step starts with looking at your own issues so that you can let go and focus on them.

14

Strategies for Older Adults and Their Caregivers

In this chapter

Growing older produces its own unique stressors both for the individual who is older and family members who serve as care providers. This chapter presents strategies for growing older healthfully. It also discusses issues and helpful techniques for adult children who must begin to provide support and care for parents, Often this need occurs before the parent is ready to admit a need for help and the situation can be painful and super stressful for all involved. This chapter shows how to apply the concepts of *CHOICES* to this stage in life.

Stop the World I Want to Get Off! This humorous title of a Broadway musical reflects a recurring human desire: When we're in a good place, we'd like to stop time and savor life. When things are going badly, we'd like to take a time out and let someone else deal with the "mess." But the milestones of life keep coming. We can't stop them. But we can master them or be mastered by them—or for most of us, get along somewhere in the middle as best we can. As we grow older, the issues may seem to take on a particularly urgent focus.

His face as red as his hair used to be, Phil was venting to me one afternoon. "What do you mean, 'Is it about them or about me?' I'm talking about my brothers, and how they treat me when they come to see Mother. They're coming again next week. I've been knocking myself out to take care of her, visiting her everyday, making the hard decisions about her medical care, riding herd on the nursing home to make sure she gets all the care she needs. And what do they do, before they even go to see her, but start in on me. Is this the right place for her? Does her care really require the expenditures I've made—and that I let them know about up front, I might add. It's pick, pick, pick—particularly about money! At this point, I feel taken advantage of and taken for granted. When they start in, I also feel a surge of the guilt I thought I'd gotten over and was okay with. I am trying to let go, and be okay, and see where they are—it really is about them, I think—but it's tough!"

Phil's mother, Eileen, who is in her late eighties, is slowly dying of the late stages of Alzheimer's dementia. Because he lives in the same town, Phil has been directly responsible for her care. Five or six years before, he was the first to notice when her short-term memory and ability to take care of her affairs began to slip, and he has been the son who has worked with his mother to make the decisions as her disease progressed. He has kept in regular e-mail touch with his two brothers. They've made a few visits, but mostly they've let him take care of matters. For a time, Eileen was able to continue to live at home with regular help, adult day care, and later a grandchild or Phil or his wife spending the nights with her. But about six or eight months before, she had moved to a nursing facility specializing in caring for persons with Alzheimer's. Phil's brothers are still having a tough time with this move.

As Phil's anger and tension began to ease, he continued to share, "They haven't seen her much. And I think they are really overwhelmed by her losses—how much she is not the person she used to be; how much she is unable to function normally and do all those little daily things we take for granted. I can remember how overwhelmed I was at first, too. I found myself continuously viewing her as she was before the onset of the illness. My long-time image of her as the mother of my youth and earlier adulthood was fixed in my mind, in my gut even. Each time I saw her I would get upset. I would weep even in her presence and then feel guilty that I was upsetting her with my tears. Since I've really examined it now, I know that deep down I wanted to be able to continue to relate to her as I had all those years, to have her respond to me as "Mom," that nurturing, interested-in-me person. That person was now gone, however, and it took time to adjust. What helped was that she quit responding to my getting upset—that forced me to step back and look at the situation and begin to accept it, to be okay.

"I don't think my brothers are yet at the acceptance stage. They are still personalizing her lack of response, her not being 'There,' and I think they are stuffing their guilt and taking it out on me. So, yes, I think it's about them. But I'm still angry at how they are shifting the blame or something onto me. I want them to simply focus on Mom, to love and support her—and me—and not be threatened by what they feel at her plight. I don't think they really care about the money—they just don't know what to do."

Phil, probably like me and many reading this book, is a member of what some have termed the "sandwich" generation. We are in our forties, fifties, and sixties, we are caring for our own children in one direction and are now having to provide more care for aging parents in the other direction. Others of you reading this book may have reached the age and circumstances where you are needing to rely more on your children or the younger generation for support, particularly if you are coping with health challenges. Or perhaps you are having to care for a spouse whose health or cognitive function is impaired. Making our way through the shifting conditions of our cherished relationships isn't easy. That's why it's tremendously important that you've developed some understanding of yourself and relationships in the ways that I've been talking about throughout this book. These understandings are tremendously important as we face aging or as you work with an aging parent. Dee is finding that to be true as she works with her mother.

Dee and her mother Marge are dealing daily with issues related to giving and receiving care. Dee is trying to bring some of the insights and skills she's been working on to her relationship with her mother and to working with her mother on how best to support her as her health has gone downhill. Over the past few years as Marge's arthritis worsened and she exercised less, she had gained a lot of weight. In addition her blood pressure had skyrocketed and heart arrhythmia problems had required a pacemaker and possibly caused small strokes. Most recently Marge has been diagnosed with breast cancer. The whole situation presents some of the toughest challenges she's ever faced, Dee says, and she knows that is even truer for her mother. Outbursts like the one that had occurred several days before are typical, she says.

CHOICES

The two of them were in Marge's kitchen. "I'm just gonna quit my pills!" Marge exclaimed in frustration—boy, was she mad! "Medicines are too expensive. This new mandated prescription drug card business doesn't make sense—it's too complicated. I've had enough. I'm too old and sick to fool with this. It's too much trouble. I'm not gonna put up with it—I'll show them who's in charge!" Today, several days later, Dee has realized that her mother had followed up on her threat and quit taking her medicines in protest.

"The most obvious problem," said Dee, "is that this reaction produced by her very real concerns and anger is understandable but not rational. Her protest is verbally directed at some 'them' she feels is responsible for 'this mess' but, of course, the only one who hears it is *me*, and she is the only one that's harmed by her leaving off her medicines. The real issue isn't the expense of the medicine—she has enough money—I think it's lack of control over her health situation and fear of gradually losing all her independence as her ability to function physically continues deteriorating. Naturally, she gets confused and depressed."

"What I need to know," Dee continued, "is how do I, as Mom's caretaker, actually take care of her? Assess what to do when she's confused and so angry? Know when to step in and take charge and when to step back? In essence, how can I make life better for her? She's facing some very severe problems. As she deteriorates, how can I best reinforce her independence and not smother her, yet be there for her and support her without making her feel too dependent? I think her fears are warping her perceptions when she gets so upset. How can I help her adjust her perception without fueling her anger? How do I make her feel secure—expand her world rather than to contract it further into isolation? How can I rally the family to support her without her feeling overwhelmed or undermined?" These are real questions that don't have easy answers.

At sometime, as one or both parents grow older, most adult children will face issues similar to Dee's or Phil's, even if our parents aren't faced with such severe health challenges. We easily recognize that as we grow from children into adults that our relationships with parents and other members of older generations are continually changing as we mature. It's often harder to understand, however, that once we reach adulthood establishing an adult relationship with our parents is not a once-for-all event that will thereafter require only minor adjustments. In actuality, those adult relationships—like any—are always changing, never static.

With modern healthcare more and more adults are living independently into their seventies, eighties and nineties. For many people, increased longevity brings an increased need for care as health issues arise (some temporary, some long-term) and as the ability to perform the daily functions of life diminishes. If you or I make it to age 65, our chances of living another 18 or 20 years is excellent. The chance of our needing some support is also excellent. Needing to face the issues of giving and receiving care is one of the byproducts of the blessing of living longer, as I look at it. So in this chapter, I'd like to offer a few brief suggestions that may help you and your family deal positively with what needs to be done.

Planning for Growing Older Healthfully

If you are thinking about your own strategies for living fully as you grow older, then my advice about many quality-of-life issues can be summed up by one simple tip: Do it before you "need" it and keep doing it. "It" covers a whole range of necessary strategies from doing the things that help you maintain your health and mobility (getting physical activity/exercise, eating heathfully, getting regular checkups, complying with treatment for any health problems), to planning for retirement and the unexpected, to dealing now with end-of-life issues (such as making a will, a living will and a durable power of attorney for health care), informing your children or other family about your plans, and so on.

Even if you must cope with some serious health issues, these conditions (even those considered life threatening) need not prevent you from *living* well. The next chapter in fact shares a number of strategies for doing just that. As we grow older, however, the reality for many of us is that we will need some support or even a great deal of support and care. Even if you have planned for long-term care, if you have children, in most instances they will want to support you and in some instances, particularly if you experience a health event that curtails your physical ability or impairs your mental function, you may need their care.

As we look toward our future, when we are in "the third half" of life (as the CarTalk brothers say of their radio show), our fear is that our children won't be as patient with us when they become caregivers as we think we were with them when they were children. Of course, deep down, our fear is that we really didn't do the best job of practicing with them the attitudes and responses that we now desire. Perhaps we *were* just a teeny, weeny bit impatient and short with them, we admit; too inclined, possibly, to show our frustration. Maybe we feel guilty about how we think we treated our own parents and are afraid that our children were watching and will treat us the same way. Or perhaps we always stressed staying strong and showing no pain while "getting on with it." Now we wonder if we'll be able to communicate our needs to our children. I've heard so many older folks who've had a major heart attack or other debilitating heart event, say "I think I'm really in trouble now—how do I look out for myself? How can I ask for help yet still stay in control of my life?"

My response is that as long as you can think for yourself— and if you're reading this book you can—it's never too late to understand yourself and to rethink your relationship with your children. You can open the doors to communication. Also the reality that you may need some assistance in daily activities or in taking care of your personal or financial affairs doesn't mean that you can't take responsibility for yourself. You can choose to live in the moment. You can choose to plan for activities that you can do and that you would like to do. For example, you can make the choice and work out the ways to stay involved in your faith community, in social and cultural events that you like, and in hobbies. You can volunteer even if you can't leave your home; for example, I know several people who are active members of their church's prayer circle, working with other committee members by phone and email and writing notes to those in their family of faith who are sick or bereaved. I've heard of another individual, who volunteers with a local agency to make daily calls to others who are alone at home to check in and make sure they are okay.

For your own care, you can work *with* your caregivers, whether they are your children or someone else, by "being okay" and opening doors to discussion and communication that they may be reluctant or unable to open. Taking these steps will "give back" to you and your children.

Issues for Adult Children in Supporting and Caring for Parents

The absolute hardest thing about providing support for our parents as they age or encounter severe, debilitating physical or cognitive problems is having to parent our parents. But one of the many benefits that you may reap from doing the work in this book is that it can help you understand yourself in relationship to your parents and the shared history that helped shape the way you connect today. Working on your own understanding can help you find the freedom you need to move beyond the bonds created by your long association with your parents to provide the best care for them while at the same time taking care of yourself.

There are a number of discoveries you may make that can help you care for your parents without going under yourself.

- You will at some level always be your parent's child even when you are "parenting" them. Recognize that they will, in all likelihood, treat you as a child, for instance, giving you instructions about how to do some task that you've been doing for years, and you may consciously have to be okay and let go the resentment you feel at their unconscious attitude.

- Recognize that the positive qualities with which you wish to support them include nurture (unconditional love) no matter what they say or do to you, support as necessary in safely performing the activities of daily living, and decision-making as necessary. The decision-making becomes hardest when a parent is no longer mentally competent to make certain decisions (such as those related to finances or understanding their medical care) but is still insisting on "doing it myself." Intervening at this point is understandably very hard but what do you do for your children? You don't let them take actions that will hurt them. At sometime you may have to do this for a parent, just as they did it for you when you were a rebellious two year old or sixteen year old.

- Because we've unconsciously granted them much of their power (in a past that we are still holding on to), even when we are adults, parents may be too powerful in their minds and ours. We must consciously choose to release that power but be okay (and not guilty) about the results.

- As they cope with physical or cognitive dysfunction, aging parents may not realize their dependence and need for care. Situations where they vehemently reject care, often irrationally, may be painful and difficult. These power issues and irrationality are always the hardest to handle. Because we love them, we don't want to hurt them emotionally; we don't want to diminish them or have them feel diminished in our eyes. When we understand in these circumstances that the issues are about them and not us, we can be okay and freed up to act rationally and lovingly even when they can't. At this point, it's very important that you see your parent where he or she really is and not where you wish he or she were. Give yourself feedback about what you are feeling and what the facts of the situation really are. Getting feedback from others involved in their care—other siblings, physicians and health care team, friends who see them regularly—can be helpful, too.

- When we understand the dynamics in our relationships with our parents, we can choose to let the guilt go. There's almost always guilt somewhere and it's always a roadblock. What's past is past. You cannot change history, but you can understand it and act positively on that understanding to create a new future. You can accept your parent where he or she is now and move ahead.

- You will understand the need for taking care of yourself so that you can give to your parent. You must have a life and appropriate boundaries. Take these reminders to heart.

- You are not a servant. It's okay to hire help. Also explore options like adult care activities.

- "Wait on" the "patient" as little as possible. Stress self-sufficiency from the beginning. If your parent is recovering from a major health problem or learning to live with the consequences, have health care services demonstrate to everyone any particular therapies, and the like. Encourage your parent to take responsibility as much as possible for him- or herself. Encourage him or her to plan activities.

- Get away; take a break. Continue to do your volunteer activities; your work; take your vacations. If your parent requires round-the-clock care, explore respite care options.

- Educate yourself about your parent's illness, but don't label. Also educate yourself about co-dependency, depression and other adjuncts to serious illness.

- Share your parents' care with your siblings, if you have some. If you are the primary caregiver and they live at a distance (or vice versa), stay in communication. As you talk together about your parents, listen to each other. Don't rush to judgment. Don't shut each other out; engage together. Joining a support group of other individuals who are caregivers can also be helpful; if you can't locate one in your community, you might want to think about organizing one.

- Prepare for dealing with negativity and irrationality. Sonya had almost given up. "Bertha, my mom, is so negative. She runs everybody off, including me and my cousins, her sister's children who live in the same town. Everything must be 'her way' or 'no way.' She picks a fight over anything and the most inane things. We have our own lives to live and jobs to maintain. And we've about had it with her." Sonya had called to check how Bertha was doing in the hospital and had just learned that she'd need surgery and Sonya's support was needed. But clearly Sonya is not prepared even to come visit, certainly not to take responsibility for her mother's care. The health care team can tell that Bertha is confused as well. They are concerned that she's not capable of managing her affairs, not just that she is a curmudgeon (which the health team also recognizes). It's never easy having to face tough circumstances such as a parent's growing mental disability or increasing negative interaction. Anticipating and planning ahead for such eventualities can help you be prepared. Sonya did eventually come for her mom's surgery and, with the support of the healthcare team, gave her mom the gift of her presence during this tough time.

- Even with the occasional mess of daily caregiving, visualize what's happened. Think about it—you've been your parent's parent. Such an act is a privilege—the culmination of life. From the sweat of your service, you've given them a gift and it can be one of life's greatest gifts to you. View it from a more distant perspective—say from three, five, or ten years from now—rather than from within the trenches. The cycle represents the fullness of growth in action as you move from parented child into adulthood, to parenthood of your own children and finally to parenting your parents. That's a Wow!

Issues for Older Adults in Supporting and Caring for Spouses

No matter how faithfully you've planned for the future as a couple, the chances are that as you grow older one partner may encounter earlier or greater health problems than the other. In my years of practice, I have seen many a wife or husband have to shoulder the responsibility of primary caregiver suddenly after a partner's abrupt illness such as an acute heart attack or stroke or more gradually as a partner's health problems grow more severe and debilitating. Planning for this possibility as a couple while you are still able is just as important as any other retirement planning.

Kitty and David were a lively couple in their seventies who loved to travel together and independently enjoyed many social activities and hobbies. On an icy day, David slipped backwards down the front steps and suffered a serious brain injury. Even with extensive rehabilitation therapy after recovery from the acute injury, David needed to use a wheelchair and required assistance with most activities of daily living. Starting from the day of the accident, Kitty threw herself 110% into caring for David. She let go all her own activities and interests and devoted herself to helping David get better.

That was all well and good during David's acute illness, but during rehab David's very astute counselor helped both partners to look more carefully and realistically at the future. Both were committed to the well-being of the other. But what would happen to them and to their relationship, asked the counselor, if Kitty totally sacrificed her life and interests to David's care? Wouldn't both grow isolated? What about Kitty's need for independence—and just as important, David's? Counseling together, the therapist helped Kitty and David see how they could rebuild the qualities they treasured in their life together in new ways. He helped them see the importance of maintaining independent lives and activities. Kitty needed to continue to have a life outside the home—to volunteer for her favorite causes and enjoy garden club, book club, and other social activities. David needed to help her do that by taking some responsibility for being independent and pursuing his interests, too. So encouraged, David soon found that he could call his own buddies and take back up the regularly morning "coffee club." His buddies didn't mind driving to the coffee shop near his house or even picking him and his wheelchair up if the weather was too bad to roll down the sidewalk.

It was hard at first for Kitty to listen to David struggle a bit on the phone (they found an amplifier helped) and she was a bit anxious the first time he motored off alone in his electric chair. But before long, they could see that making sure that both of them had a life was also promoting their sense of well-being and health. Being as active as possible was actually helping David improve his functional abilities.

What Kitty and David would say to other couples who find themselves in situations where one spouse must be the primary caregiver for the other is that whether you are "caregiver" or "cared for," take responsibility for yourself and make sure you "have a life."

CHOICES

The tips I gave earlier for children providing care for their adult parents works well for spouses caring for their partners.

A Final Word

Books can be, and have been, written on the art of caregiving. This chapter has shared just a few brief thoughts on very complex issues and circumstances. There are now a number of useful resources available on the Internet. Here are a few good resources.

www.familycaregiver.org The National Family Caregivers Association provides links to many resources

www.caregiver.org The Family Caregiver Alliance has numerous factsheets and caregiver guides

www.familycaregiving101.org A Web-based guide from the National Family Caregivers Association and the National Alliance for Caregiving

www.positiveaging.org Positive Aging Resource Center has tips for dealing with life changes, staying connected, promoting health, and caregiving.

www.alzheimers.org ADEAR, the Alzheimer's Disease Education & Referral Center from the National Institute on Aging, has a number of publications and resources related to caring for individuals with dementia.

15
You've Been There—So What's Next?

In this chapter

Often it takes a health crisis or diagnosis to wake us up to the need for change. No matter how serious the problem, it can be a motivator and a breakthrough to a new, fulfilling life. The event might be as traumatic as a heart attack or diagnosis of cancer. Or maybe the tests have come back positive for diabetes or chronic obstructive pulmonary disease. It's never too late to choose freedom and a fully realized life. You are not your disease. This chapter presents seven steps for choosing a new life even when faced with what may seem a life-threatening challenge.

It's Never Too Late—Using Health Problems as a Stepping Stone to New Life

Henrietta was brought to the Emergency Department by the EMTs. Because she was so upset and anxious, they were about to restrain her. Her implanted defibrillator had fired for the fourth time that week. Naturally, she was frightened for her life. The rescue team had found her stable but in serious need of professional reassurance. In the past four years she had endured numerous cardiovascular problems: blood clots in her legs and lungs, a heart attack and heart failure, then the complication of a pacemaker and defibrillator (she had already survived cancer ten years earlier). In spite of her familiarity with medical procedures, the need for the pacemaker/

defibrillator had occurred so quickly that Retty hadn't had time to be educated about all the important aspects. Of course, she knew the defibrillator offered her condition a better life-preserving option than medicines; however, she didn't really expect it to go off and hit her so hard, not four times in one week! She just wanted the whole problem fixed, once and for all. The jubilance of the emergency staff really bothered her.

"They think they're so cute telling me I'm fine and congrat-ulating me that I'm still alive. That doesn't help me in the moment after I'm shocked—when my adrenalin's pumping and I'm so upset—trying to collect myself again. Yes, they give me security, but they seem to enjoy themselves too much. This is supposed to be about me. The way they act makes me not tell them how I really feel."

Henrietta felt buffeted about. She was ready to try anything, including a fairly risky surgical procedure that might correct the underlying rhythm problem the defibrillator was responding to. Making that decision restored her feeling of calm and eased her anxiety, even though she understood that the short-term risk was greater than that posed by the defibrillator.

Contrast Henrietta's story with Joe's. Joe has suffered bouts of cardiac chest pains for six months. Although his coronary plaque has required balloon angioplasty with stent placement, he has not had a heart attack. Physically, Joe is in good shape over all and has taken the right steps to manage his heart disease and perhaps even improve his condition. His prognosis is good; at present he does not have a particularly high risk for a heart event. But he's a basket case—scared to death that something unexpected will take him out. That's what happened to his dad and several other relatives in his childhood—no warning, then—boom—they were gone. These early experiences no doubt feed Joe's extreme anxiety and distress. When he does have to visit the doctor, particularly when he must undergo testing, he manifests severe signs of distress—racing pulse, more chest pain, skyrocketing blood pressure, huddling on the exam table. But he goes.

Finally, let's consider Yancy, who's had a huge heart attack, has a defibrillator implanted and currently has heart failure. Yet Yancy will admit to no stress. He just ignores his heart condition and gets on with doing his work. He's the president and chairman of a large business that employs three thousand and does forty percent of its business with government—big business. Blindness to the inherent stress of his work and its effects upon his body is an issue that Yancy needs to face—in fact, it's a matter of life and death. But for the moment, he's blind to his blindness, not to mention deaf to the entreaties of his family and advice of his physicians.

Each of these three individuals is grappling with major health issues. To a marked degree, all three are reacting to the stress of their situations (which they may not see as stress), rather than understanding that they are stressed and choosing positive behaviors that will help them release the stress, rather than "stuff" it. What are the impediments to change for these individuals? Can they choose to change? Yes. Is it too late? No. It's never too late. Let's remember —our goal is to make the most of living.

Life—Choose It! Reach for It!

Life's a vision. Change is a vision. Focus is a vision. Strength and values are visions. Going to the moon for the first time, back in the sixties, started with a vision. Sure it took a lot of planning and work to land a man on the moon's surface. But the reality started with the vision. You and I are able to reach for life, to choose a life worth living and to make it a reality—no matter what our health challenges. Our success starts with vision. Then, as the Beatles sang, we'll need "a little help" from our friends.

After a heart event or other life-changing health crisis, people who do well typically pause and "step back" and look at the bigger picture. They focus and refocus on "what is"—they learn the facts about their disease. They accept these facts as an empowering foundation to move forward from. They examine and make use of healthful, protective boundaries (not isolating armor). Then they focus and envision the future; they choose life. If you are facing major or catastrophic health issues, this positive approach can work for you, too.

You are not your disease

If you've had a heart attack or cancer or a stroke, or another bad health event, the old *you* is not the same. You can never go back. That old *you* is gone forever. That's a fact that must be accepted. You can grieve for that self—a little grief is appropriate—but you can't resurrect the self you were before. Nor should you wish to. You must move on—face forward, not backward, and envision the new *you*. So you see, accepting the facts does not equal giving up. You are not your disease. Repeat that right now: "I am not my disease." That also is a fact. Don't you forget—or let anyone else forget it.

You'll need the support of others; that support is lifesaving. But you may need to choose those supporters who are willing to follow your lead of looking forward, going forward. You and those who care about you need first to accept that life will not be the same—you can never go back to being the *old you*. But you can make the *new you* come to life. That *new you* can and will incorporate all that's positive from the *old you*. You must grow through the events and live on—move on. You will need to educate yourself about your condition so that you can be an equal partner in your care with your physicians. The more you understand about your condition the easier it is to carry out your physicians' treatment recommendations such as taking medications, getting the right exercise or physical therapy, or following the right diet. But the most important step, starts with your vision. You need help from others, but you are the only one who can come up with your vision for yourself and your future. You will find that accepting the facts brings you a peace and power to go forward to discover all the new opportunities that await. This is a recommitment that you need to make daily.

Help me to change

Ed asked me for a brief appointment after support group one evening. Later in my office, he poured out his thoughts.

"I don't want to go through the heart attack or another intervention again. Since I was ill, I'm experiencing a sensitivity that somehow is comforting. Though I felt comfortable with myself before the experience, I don't want to go back to that old self because I know I was blind to so many things. Instead, I want to grow and carry those experiences with me. I now know my present health is a result of my past and I now know it'll be best for me to go forward, as a changed person—and I want that—I want to live! I want better health in order to enjoy my family and see my children and grandchildren grow up—to enjoy life. I've heard the instructions and taken the 'course' on making better choices and developing a new mindset, but where do I hit 'enter' – how do I do it – how do I actually change? Though I'm a believer that I need to change, I need help getting where I know I need to be—where I want to be."

"I am now at the place you wanted me to be—on my knees pleading for help. And now you say it's up to me, for if I have a burning desire to change, I'll find a way. You repeatedly tell me you'll be there for me to help me to change. I say again—I am the one who wants to change. Because I have a different outlook, I'm asking myself, what have I done to all those I've influenced—my family—my wife and my children? Can I be a better influence now, help establish better communication and happier, more fulfilling relationships? I really want to change—even if it takes me the rest of my life to do it. I want something better than running from the fear of the inevitable—death. I want to enjoy, to be fulfilled in pursuing this life and fold it into the one beyond—to eventually approach it with a peace in my mind because I've changed and given my best – contributed to those I influence, love and care about. Can you help me?"

Ed is ready to move on, to create his vision. He has accepted the facts about his health condition and educated himself about the best medical and physical treatments. But now he wants to find new ways of relating to his loved ones and work to deal with all the stresses of life.

All the ideas and techniques in this book are valid for Ed and for you. They provide all the clues, keys, and techniques you need to envision new ways of living based on new ways of relating to your life and the others in it. But I'd like to highlight a few points just for you.

- Know yourself.
- Take responsibility
- Catch the vision of a new life.
- Find a coach
- Work as a partner with your doctor(s)
- Comply with your treatment plan
- Plan for the future
- Quit looking over your shoulder and live!

First, know yourself. Narrow your focus deep inside yourself. Only in this way will you broaden your scope to reach out to others—from self to others. So follow the poet's advice, "To thine ownself be true."

We learn a view of ourselves from others from infancy forward. How do you see yourself? Do you have labels either you or others have assigned to you? If so, identify them and change your labels. When we change, we have to let something go. To repeat, when we change, we have to let something go.

We learn guilt, too. Our guilt is passed down—it's something we're taught. Ed's mother suffers with progressive dementia; her deteriorating condition has taught him about letting go the urge to control—being okay with his helplessness to aid her. Being okay means he has let go his guilt and the stress produced by that guilt. As a result, he no longer feels obligated (like a prison sentence) to visit his mother daily, especially since she doesn't recognize him or remember him or his visits. He doesn't have to defend or explain to himself why he isn't visiting more—there's nothing he can do. With this burden removed, however, he now wants to visit, but only because he loves her—she's his mom. (Take note: it appears the one who previously taught the guilt is now teaching it's okay to let it go and to simply be.) It's alright for you to be okay with your health event. What happened, happened. What is, is. You must also forgive yourself for any ways you think you may have contributed to your health difficulties. But where you go next is your choice.

In order to change, we have to know more about ourselves. Support groups of people who've had similar health experiences can help you better understand what dealing with the disease is like and also help you to sort out your feelings about your condition and the changes it's bringing to your life. Discovering self and others is a growth process—the path is circular and spiral—from one to and through the other. It's orderly, not chaotic, but it may be leisurely, not speedy. Give yourself room to breathe, to think.

Take responsibility. You now know that influential others played a big part in your life's development, and now as an adult, you must take over, take on, and take back all those responsibilities. You must be accountable to yourself—turn yourself around—and change. Both your motivation for change and your resistance to that change are working for and against you. Yet these forces taken together are not just part of the problem but also part of the solution. Take note—in your strengths lie the answers to your weaknesses and vulnerabilities. You must get to know yourself beneath your superficial cover—and while there, specifically focus on your anger, internal rages (yes, especially at what's happened to your health), and other generators of unhealthy behaviors. Explore yourself in order to get to all the hurts and fears you've experienced, in order to understand them and transform them. Because various angers mask what's really going on, anger serves as a poor compensation. Anger—"rage, rage against the dying of the light" the poet said—may not be the best choice in the case of severe health problems if the anger consists of reactions that continuously accumulate and contribute to illness. Being determined to fight back, taking reasoned steps, and living optimistically even with bulldog stubbornness can be positive in ways that unfocused anger or even rage at the disease cannot.

I like to remind patients that this is a commitment to yourself that you need to renew every morning. This is a very positive thing you can do for yourself. As a person of faith, I like to use a favorite line from the *Psalms* that keeps me focused on the positive of what I'm doing for myself and those I care about: "This is the day which the Lord has made. Let us rejoice and be glad in it."

Catch the vision: To change, see yourself as changed and take charge of yourself. When you've caught the vision, keep it in front of you. It's clear you do want to change and you need to see that decision in action. Therefore, envision yourself as successful, the way you want to be. Consider the ways you label and see yourself. If these views aren't helpful or factual today, change them—make them right—be true to your self and to your foundational values. If you slip into old patterns, don't kick yourself. Instead, acknowledge what happened, examine the causes, be okay, and go forward. Never use one slip, or two, as an easy excuse to quit.

Two people who have shared their stories with the larger community strike me as powerful examples of how you can take charge and see yourself as changed, as the new you. And choose to go there.

John Nash, the brilliant Nobel Laureate in mathematics, suffered much of his adult life from schizophrenia, yet he was able, with the understanding and unfailing support of his wife and friends, to shape a productive life and use his gifts. His story was the subject of the film *A Beautiful Mind*.

Reynolds Price, the imminent novelist, poet, playwright and Duke professor, was at the height of his career, when a colleague noticed that as he walked, one foot dragged slightly. Tests revealed an extremely rare spinal cancer that had wrapped itself all around his spinal column. Almost miraculous surgery removed the cancer, but Price suffered inordinately with paralysis of his lower body, constant overwhelming pain, prolonged hospitalizations, and learning to live with radical lifestyle changes. Even after his body tissues had long recovered from the surgeries, the chronic pain raged on. Various pain control drug regimens dulled the agony some, but also dulled Price's creative mind. Throughout the struggle he kept working, kept creating.

Finally, after many trials and errors, with the help of a creative group of pain management specialists, Reynolds Price found new ways to understand the pain and to use his mind to control its effect. His story, which he shared in his book, *A Whole New Life,* is riveting; and I recommend it to anyone dealing with life-changing illness. Price looked squarely at all the facts and issues, and with help, found the balance that would enable him to create a new and fulfilling life. I think his writing for the rest of his life was more powerful than ever.

To change, one needs a coach. Even though we're adults, it's always helpful to have companionship—a mentor—not to carry you, but to provide support. A coach can also be a helpful mirror, reflecting what you need to see and hear. Of course, you've proved many times that you can successfully carry out specific tasks and jobs on your own. But a catastrophic illness is a huge blow. The expression "crash and burn" comes to mind for emotional impact. At such times we often need a coach again. Support groups of people with similar conditions can be very helpful as can informal visits with others who have "walked in your shoes." Don't let false pride get in your way of taking advantage of these opportunities.

Open yourself up to your loved ones, too. Change comes best in an environment of clear connection between individuals. The atmosphere is clearer because of two-way communications, free of confusion. Of course, environmental circumstances change and negative things may happen, but love is the spark that kindles the hope—gives the joy and gratitude, keeping the spirit alive in both good and difficult times.

Work as a partner with your doctor(s). If you are grappling with a serious illness or health condition, you can do more to promote positive outcomes by working as a partner with your doctor. If you see yourself as "partner" not "patient" and co-equal in the relationship, then you can foster a good working relationship with your physician, even if he or she doesn't take the same attitude.

You may have wondered, as you headed toward an appointment, does the doctor actually need my help? The answer is *yes*. There's more to a productive visit than merely showing up with insurance cards in hand, voicing the problem and asking what the doctor is going to do toward improving or solving your problem. It's important for you to be involved because it's your problem—you're the one "bleeding." Even the most perceptive physician will fall short of adequate discovery of your problem unless you share clues and lend a hand. In addition, the assessment and treatment programs won't work without your understanding, ownership and action. So, besides showing up for your appointment, what homework can you do to better prepare for visits with your physicians—whether the visit is a first-time evaluation with a new specialist or the umpteenth follow-up with your long-time doctor?

CHOICES

One of the most important things you can do is to take a minute to describe to yourself what messages you want your doctor to hear—the bottom-line messages—given in simple terms and without so many qualifying details. Think about this ahead of time, so you can choose your words. You might even jot a few points down so you'll remember to share them. Then allow the physician to ask pertinent questions for better medical understanding toward a clearer diagnosis (since the proper diagnosis determines the work-up and the treatment).

The next step is to prepare a list of concerns and questions you have thought through for presentation to your doctor. Write these down, too. Hand your doctor a copy to review on the spot and ask pointed and clarifying questions so as to process them as quickly as possible. The other thing to consider is whether you want your doctor to take what you say at face value or decode you. Because we all have our own unique method of interacting with those who know us, it may be difficult for us to change our behavior. All too often, we expect those who know us to decode our behaviors rather than being sure to give them a clear indication of what we are feeling. But if you will consciously think about the information or feelings that you want to share with the physician and then try to share them clearly, I can promise you that your efforts will improve the level of communication and provide an opportunity for a more efficient and effective visit.

Besides these suggestions, which other responsibilities belong to you and which to your physicians? Every doctor's intent is usually to be helpful; however, it's your life and your problem. After all, who's taking care of whom? Aren't you able to work toward bringing yourself up to speed—to research your issues to be as informed as possible, to be responsible for yourself, to find out what you're to do to maximize your health—and then do it? Yes, you are able and capable to rise above your issues to improve your health and to do more than get by or just survive.

Comply with your treatment plan. If you have worked with your doctors as partners, then you should understand your options for treatment and have played a part in choosing or confirming the steps you will undertake, the medicines, the therapies, and so forth. Now it's your job to follow through. You can choose to do it. If you run into difficulties, act like the partner with your physician that you aim to be. If I had a dollar for every time a patient said, for instance, "Oh, I didn't like the way those blood pressure pills made me feel, so I just quit taking them," I'd have a very hefty nestegg. For most conditions (like high blood pressure) there are multiple treatment options, so tell your physician if you run into problems, and keep pursuing options, don't just cop out—it's too risky.

If you have problems finding more information or following through on treatment plans, ask your physician for help. Ask particularly if you have difficulty with any of the prescribed treatment regimens (including physical activity/therapy, diet, weight loss efforts, medications, etc.); be honest with your physicians about those difficulties. They can help you make adjustments or find support to make those changes. Above all, remember it's your life and it's in your control—you are to partner with your doctor(s) in working for the outcomes you want. In our haste and habits, we physicians sometimes are as guilty of labeling as anyone else— thinking of patients or cases or "beds" rather than individuals—but if you refuse to live down to those labels and claim your role as partner, most physicians will respond in ways that you will find supportive and helpful.

Plan for the future. All of us do ourselves and family a favor when we plan for the future. But planning for the future can bring even more peace of mind if you are living with a serious health condition. Failure to plan puts you or family members in the position of having to react, rather than respond, should you have an acute or catastrophic event related to your health condition.

One afternoon I received an urgent call from the distressed daughter of Julie, a vibrant, active lady of eighty-two, whom I'd known for nearly twenty-five years. Her daughter was calling from the hospital where Julie had been taken with a serious heart attack. At the moment Julie was unconscious and on life support; her prognosis was poor. Given the impact of the heart attack, the attending hospital physicians felt she had little chance of living and recovering and gently advised removing life support. Julie's daughter was upset and in a quandary. What should she do? Her mother had not prepared a living will, but she had talked to her daughter about her wishes. As we talked quietly, I was able to help the daughter remember what Julie had said she wanted in just such circumstances. The daughter and I also had information about Julie that the hospital team did not have. We knew that she was very active, faithfully following an exercise program and healthy diet; we knew that physically, if she survived the heart attack, she had a better chance of a good functional recovery than the care team might suppose. Julie's daughter knew that if there was a good chance of such a functional recovery her mother would want to pursue aggressive treatment. Even though Julie had not made a living will or detailed plans, her conversations with her daughter provided the basis the daughter needed to tell the doctors to continue treatment. She had also called on me for a medical opinion because I knew her mother. Within 24 to 48 hours, Julie's body began to respond to the treatment. As soon as she was conscious, her "fighting spirit" also showed through. A few weeks later, Julie walked into my office with a big smile, a hug and a thank you. She has a few limitations that she didn't have earlier and a stricter regimen, but she's glad to be alive—she has more to give, she says, and she's glad that she's alive to be able to keep on giving.

Are there points of no return? What can you do about that?

When you are diagnosed with a serious illness, such as heart disease or a cancer, your first thought may be, is this the end? Later as you manage your condition or struggle to do so, you may find yourself wondering if there's a point of no return for making change? Physically? Emotionally?

Yes. There are possible points of no return in every life and probably with every serious or life-threatening health condition. Because they are there, however, doesn't mean that you have to go past one. Being aware of the dangers can help you use possible points of no return as motivators—as points of new return, if you will.

Judy's experience, for me, is a story of lost opportunity. From at least middle-age on she experienced one serious health problem after another. In one sense, she was a "survivor." In another sense, she was a "loser" because she missed so many opportunities to turn around and live more healthfully and fully.

As a so-called sickly child, Judy had been labeled as "frail" and was continually spoiled and allowed tons of slack. The world revolved around her. As an adult, she continued to demand slack and spoiling. As a wife and parent, she controlled the family so that her needs were indulged first. She had never been required to exert any self-discipline as a child or adolescent and she consequently lacked self-awareness, self-discipline and a sense of personal accountability as an adult. She was unable to see problems coming when they were small blips on the horizon or even when they grew larger. She was never able to make appropriate changes and move out of the way.

When she developed high blood pressure and chronic bronchitis, she procrastinated. When her physicians told her that she needed to stop smoking and to eat more healthfully and exercise moderately in order to control her health conditions, she resisted. No, she said, she didn't want to make changes, she didn't have to make changes.

Her high blood pressure continued out of control along with her two-pack-a-day cigarette habit. At age 62, she suffered a stroke. She was forced to quit smoking for a while, but then went back to it. A decade later, she developed lung cancer. She endured multiple surgeries and radiation treatments. But again she made no lifestyle changes. Because she grew weaker, she fell often. But she would not eat properly and would not perform the prescribed physical therapy to strengthen her muscles. Instead, she demanded a return to her old life. But physical weakness and malnutrition were soon followed by mental confusion. At this point Judy passed the absolute point of no return. She had had many wake-up calls in her life and many opportunities to choose change, but she stubbornly refused each.

Judy's biggest problems were not really physical but attitudinal. Anyone can choose to live fully even in the face of catastrophic illness. Sometimes that living fully means making peace with the prospect of death, accepting the facts, and then turning to enjoying your family and life as fully as possible. Such habits established as early as possible in life lay a foundation most people can rely on when life deals out the hardest blows.

Are there points of no return? Yes. But if you are prepared mentally, you can choose to go forward with life. Because she would not examine her life and choices, the circumstances controlled Judy.

A Simple Story

Always remember in every thing that you are *you*—a person of worth and value. Claim that dignity and don't let go. And what you claim for yourself, grant to others. You may even need to remind them from time to time. One of my younger colleagues recently rediscovered the value of this mindset.

As I was making rounds at the hospital one morning, Susan waylaid me. "Why on earth are you treating 'Bed 22' so aggressively, when all her problems predict that she won't do well and may well die. Why put her through all that?" Susan's tone was emphatic and she was just warming up when she was paged to respond to another patient. I was okay with Susan's concern, because I knew that she truly was considering the patient's need—but I did disagree with her because I knew "Bed 22" as Patricia and knew her wishes about what kind of measures she wanted taken if a crisis arose. When I checked back on Patricia that afternoon, Susan again spotted me and flagged me down, this time with an apology. It seems that between morning and afternoon, she had discovered that "Bed 22" was a person she knew, "Aunt Patty," a dear, kind aunt of one of her best friends from high school. Susan was surprised at her own about-face—now she wanted the health care team to do as much as possible to treat Aunt Patty.

So never forget, you are a person of value. Don't forget that about your family and your health care team—don't let them forget it about you. The best way to do that is to be proactive in your own care and planning and to work with your family and your health care team as a partner, not a patient.

Quit Looking Over Your Shoulder and Live!

And now what?
- Redefine health for yourself.
- Have no guilt for your past and be open to change.

- You're in control and healthy options are the ultimate choice, whatever your health.
- Emphasize education about your health and illness.
- Learn to adjust (as soon and fast as possible).
- Seek coaching (especially with your doctor) to facilitate the process for better understanding where you stand, what your options are for action and going forward, essentially, giving-in and being totally involved in the process rather than giving-up.

As in a sport, where we practice and practice the fundamentals, we may later realize that we enjoyed the exercise in and of itself, for when engaged with a real opponent in a game situation we find it's harder to control ourselves and the opponent. We often tend to focus on the rigidity of the practice situation rather than putting it all together. After the basics are set and rote, forget practice except to stay in shape and simply play to the best of your ability, no more rehearsing. We can't do both at the same time, for they require different mind-sets.

We're learning to focus and at times, to refocus—adjusting our mind-set to get the most out of our situation. Said another way, to focus on the practice, we aren't staying in the game and moving according to where the ball is and what our opponent is doing. It's at that point that we have to meld all we know and all our practice together, refocus and live (or continuing the sport analogy), just play ball.

And so it is with our lives. We're developing a mind-set to guide us in and through life, no matter what. And don't keep looking over your shoulder or waiting for the second shoe to drop; don't look back, it's not helpful, except in a historical sense. The mindset takes its lead from our goals and values for living, not what's surrounding us. Though our surroundings need attention, at times it may only be a distraction to deal with or an excuse to drift focus off-course.

On the other hand, our focus may guide us to do nothing, to sit still, rest and "smell the roses" and not become absorbed in the distraction, for in the moment it's not important. This effort is about you, about protecting and preserving your health. About opening your mind and helping you hurdle the stumbling blocks. About doing all needed for health, visualizing the healthiest life you can live. Then, with maintaining that in mind, live life to the fullest. In this river of life, the current continually moves, so if you want to grow, you have to keep stroking to move forward or you go backwards and essentially loose.

Make Use of Your Working Skill-Sets in Everyday Life

After a stellar professional career, Beth had recently retired. She had been aware of the looming change coming but thought she could deal with it and make plans for the rest of her life when her job was completed. One morning soon after retiring, she woke up before dawn feeling the windblast of change, couldn't catch her breath, and felt panicky. She initially brushed it off as anxiety, which she had previously experienced; however, after the sensation of a weight descended on her chest with noticeable, perfuse sweating, she reconsidered and called 911. Our team was introduced to her on discharge day after her small heart attack, which resulted in the placement of two coronary stents. She elected to enter the support group as part of the cardiac rehab program.

Over the first few visits, she shared the story of her heart event and vigorously entered in the discussions. On the next visit, she shared having been a childhood victim of sexual abuse. She thought she had pretty much resolved the many issues associated with the abuse since she eventually could discuss the abuse freely and chose not to engage in counseling or formal therapy. She noted being more assertive than her younger brother and defended both of them, the protector against onslaughts from the parents. She married, had no children and divorced her husband because of his alcoholism and verbal abuse. All these experiences she felt were tangible evidence that she had resolved the abuse problem and was able to take care of herself. Wrong thinking.

In the beginning, we discussed thinking. There are many kinds of thinking: logical, situational, critical, magical and wrong. Much wrong thinking comes from internal processing that generates the messages we respond to. As a result these messages and voices come in many forms and disguises. We need to be familiar with those voices and sort the valued ones from the trash, the ones that are from pure illusions in our pasts. It's up to us to prune them for if they risk getting us in trouble or influence us to make bad choices, we can no longer afford the consequences they bring and must let them go. It's our life and now we're driving, we're in charge and are responsible for ourselves.

Beth knew she had many powerful work skills as a leader, teacher and counselor besides the expertise associated with her profession. She was gifted both technically and as a people-person. But she had buried, unacknowledged issues that were essentially blocking any connection between her two worlds, the successful one at work and her unspoken sense of failure on the personal side. Her unresolved defense burdens were blocking her from processing her abuse history to a more comfortable level that included freedom from the unapparent weight of that abuse. Once she looked realistically at these unacknowledged burdens she realized a sense of freedom and a sense that her future held the promise of normal interpersonal relationships beyond work.

In group, we asked her to consider shifting her working skill-sets, those gifts that had been an integral part of her success, over to her personal and family life. It was amazing that she made the shift so easily and successfully. She confidently entered therapy to continue the much needed processing. She was reinforced from both fronts, from a huge celebration of appreciation given by her previous employer, accompanied by many awards of service, and from the rehab group. She and extended family were pleased to see her energized self re-emerge.

We can each bring all our skill-sets to the table of life and use them to enrich the experience and to ensure we do our part to bring out everybody's best, for all to gain. This means we make use of all the tools in our repertoire that make us who we are, including those used at work and at play. We need to bring them home to serve the people we care most about. Influencing them at the heart of the family can affect generations to come.

This freedom means we'll finally accept ourselves as who we are. It's okay to keep honing our skill-sets even after our jobs end, to refresh the habit of solution-solving-thinking to be more aware of the "wrong" types of thinking that block our progress to the freedom of streams of clear thinking. Additionally, we can use our memories to engage encounters with encouraging mentors who reinforced clear thinking and were examples of characteristics we want to master for a life lived to the fullest. It's also okay to patiently practice delaying immediate gratification. What we're doing by continuous patience and thinking is to learn to be smarter than and stay a step ahead of our internal desires that so often get us off-track and stumble into trouble.

Such actions give us hope. Our hope is in our new awareness, in the renewed ability to focus and refocus, in untethered and unburdened freedom of choice, in improved thinking, in continuously honing our skills, in developing and having broader connections, in thankfulness, in our newly discovered selves and in our Maker. Regrettably, there's no quick fix. Therefore, "guard your *heart*—(for) it's the wellspring of life." This concept and advice is well said, for in Biblical terms, the heart is "the center of the human spirit, from which spring emotions, thought, motivations, courage and action" (NIV). So, think and rethink your mindset, make better choices because of it and live on with a peace that you're improving your health and doing your best; and remember we're all works in progress.

Selected Resources

The resources provided on these pages include books and scientific journal articles with background information or more extensive information on many of the topics and issues discussed in CHOICES. Resources are presented in chronological order, starting with the most recent publications.

USEFUL WEBSITES

American Heart Association: www.heart.org

American College of Cardiology
      Cardiosource website: www.cardiosource.org
      CardioSmart website: www.cardiosmart.org

American College of Physicians
    Resource pages for Patients and Families
www.acponline.org/patients_families/

American Psychological Association Psychology Help Center
www.apa.org/helpcenter/index.aspx

Centers for Disease Control and Prevention: www.cdc.gov

www.MedlinePlus.gov   A source of evidence-based health information for consumers.

www.mayoclinic.com   A source of reliable health information provided by the physicians and health care professionals of the Mayo Clinic.

Sharecare: www.sharecare.com
    An interactive platform that shares expert health information and allows you to ask questions and get answers from health professionals.

BOOKS AND JOURNAL ARTICLES

Anger and Anger Management

Books

Williams, Redford, MD, and Virginia Williams PhD. *Anger Kills: Seventeen Strategies for Controlling the Hostility that Can Harm Your Health.* New York: HarperPerrenial, 1994.

Journal Articles

Smith TW, Uchino BN, Berg CA, Florsheim P. Marital discord and coronary artery disease: a comparison of behaviorally defined discrete groups. Journal of Consulting and Clinical Psychology. 2012 Feb;80(1):87-92.

Newman JD, Davidson KW, Shaffer JA, Schwartz JE, Chaplin W, Kirkland S, Shimbo D. Observed hostility and the risk of incident ischemic heart disease: a prospective population study from the 1995 Canadian Nova Scotia Health Survey. Journal of the American College of Cardiology. 2011 Sep 13;58(12):1222-8.

Haukkala A, Konttinen H, Laatikainen T, Kawachi I, Uutela A. Hostility, anger control, and anger expression as predictors of cardiovascular disease. Psychosomatic Medicine. 2010 Jul;72(6):556-62.

Anxiety and Depression

Books

Beck, Aaron T., MD, and Brad A. Alford, PhD. *Depression: Causes and Treatment.* 2nd edition. Philadelphia, PA: University of Pennsylvania Press, 2009.

Miller, Mark D, MD, and Charles F. Reynolds III, MD. *Depression and Anxiety in Later Life: What Everyone Needs to Know.* Baltimore, Maryland: The Johns Hopkins University Press, 2012.

Journal Articles

Valkanova V, Ebmeier KP. Vascular risk factors and depression in later life: A systematic review and meta-analysis. Biological Psychiatry. 2012; Dec 10. [epub ahead of print].

Davidson KW. Depression and coronary heart disease. ISRN Cardiology.2012; Nov 22. [epub ahead of print]

Pizzi C, Santarella L, Costa MG, Manfrini O, Flacco ME, Capasso L, Chiarini S, Di Baldassarre A, Manzoli L. Pathophysiological mechanisms linking depression and atherosclerosis: an overview. Journal of Biological Regulators and Homeostatic Agents. 2012 Oct-Dec;26(4):775-82.

Zunszain PA, Hepgul N, Pariante CM. Inflammation and depression. Current Topics in Behavioral Neurosciences. 2012; May 3. [epub ahead of print]

Behavior and Neurobiology

Books
McEwen, B.S. *The End of Stress as We Know It.* New York: Dana Press, 2002 (Available as an e-book.)

Journal Articles

Muscatell KA, Eisenberger NI. A social neuroscience perspective on stress and health. Social and Personality Psychological Compass. 2012 Dec 1;6(12):890-904.

McEwen BS Brain on stress: How the social environment gets under the skin Proceedings Of The National Academy of Sciences of The United States Of America 2012 Oct 16; 109:17180-17185.

McEwen BS The ever-changing brain: Cellular and molecular mechanisms for the effects of stressful experiences. Developmental Neurobiology 2012 Jun;72(6):878-890.

McEwen, B.S. and Stellar, E. Stress and the individual: mechanisms leading to disease. *Archives of Internal Medicine 1993;* 153:2093-2101.

McEwen, B.S. Protective and damaging effects of stress mediators. New England Journal of Medicine 1998; 338: 171-179.

McEwen, B.S. Stress, adaptation, and disease: Allostasis and allostatic load. *Annals of the New York Academy of Science 1998;* 840:33-44.

Cardiovascular Disease, Risk Factors

Books

Allan, Robert, MD, and Jeffrey Fisher, MD, eds.. *Heart and Mind: The Practice of Cardiac Psychology.* Second edition. APA Books, 2011.

Fuster, Valentin MD, PhD. with Joseph Corbella. *The Heart Manual.* New York: Harper, 2010.

Journal Articles

Boehm JK, Kubzansky LD. The heart's content: the association between positive psychological well-being and cardiovascular health. Psychological Bulletin 2012 Jul;138(4):655-91.

Low CA, Thurston RC, Matthews KA. Psychosocial factors in the development of heart disease in women: current research and future directions. Psychosomatic Medicine 2010 Nov;72(9):842-54.

Albus C. Psychological and social factors in coronary heart disease. Annals of Medicine 2010 Oct;42(7):487-94.

Hamer M, Malan L. Psychophysiological risk markers of cardiovascular disease. Neuroscience and Biobehavioral Reviews 2010 Sep;35(1):76-83.

Franklin BA. Impact of psychosocial risk factors on the heart: changing paradigms and perceptions. The Physician and Sportsmedicine 2009 Oct;37(3):35-7.

Endothelial Dysfunction in Heart Disease and Other Chronic Diseases

Books

Shauna, Dauphinee and Aly Karsan, Eds. *Endothelial Dysfunction and Inflammation.* Series: Progress in Inflammation Research. New York: Springer Publishing Company, 2010.

De Caterina, Raffaele and Peter Libby, Eds. *Endothelial Dysfunctions in Vascular Disease.* Malden, MA: Blackwell, 2007.

Journal Articles

Solini A, Stea F, Santini E, Bruno RM, Duranti E, Taddei S, Ghiadoni L. Adipocytokine levels mark endothelial function in normotensive individuals. Cardiovascular Diabetology 2012 Aug 31;11(1):103.

Bruno RM, Ghiadoni L, Seravalle G, Dell'oro R, Taddei S, Grassi G. Sympathetic regulation of vascular function in health and disease. Frontiers in Physiology 2012;3:284.

Virdis A, Bruno RM, Neves MF, Bernini G, Taddei S, Ghiadoni L. Hypertension in the elderly: an evidence-based review. Current Pharmaceutical Design 2011;17(28):3020-31.

Versari D, Daghini E, Virdis A, Ghiadoni L, Taddei S. Endothelial dysfunction as a target for prevention of cardiovascular disease. Diabetes Care 2009 Nov;32 Suppl 2:S314-21.

Versari D, Daghini E, Virdis A, Ghiadoni L, Taddei S. The ageing endothelium, cardiovascular risk and disease in man. Experimental Physiology 2009 Mar;94(3):317-21.

Inflammation, Role in Cardiovascular and Other Chronic Diseases

Books

Wick, Georg and Cecilia Grundtman, Eds. *Inflammation and Atherosclerosis.* New York: Springer Publishing Company, 2012.

Serhan, Charles N, Peter A Ward, Derek W. Gilroy, Eds. *Fundamentals of Inflammation.* Cambridge, UK: Cambridge University Press, 2010.

Journal Articles

Gouin JP, Glaser R, Malarkey WB, Beversdorf D, Kiecolt-Glaser J. Chronic stress, daily stressors, and circulating inflammatory markers. Health Psychology 2012 Mar;31(2):264-8.

Rooks C, Veledar E, Goldberg J, Bremner JD, Vaccarino V. Early trauma and inflammation: role of familial factors in a study of twins. Psychosomatic Medicine 2012 Feb-Mar;74(2):146-52.

Cardiovascular Disease

Libby P. Inflammation in atherosclerosis. Arteriosclerosis, Thrombosis, and Vascular Biology 2012 Sep;32(9):2045-51.

Chiang JJ, Eisenberger NI, Seeman TE, Taylor SE. Negative and competitive social interactions are related to heightened proinflammatory cytokine activity. Proceedings of the National Academy of Sciences of the U S A. 2012 Feb 7;109(6):1878-82.

Packard RR, Libby P. Inflammation in atherosclerosis: from vascular biology to biomarker discovery and risk prediction. Clinical Chemistry 2008 Jan;54(1):24-38.

Appels A, Bär FW, Bär J, Bruggeman C, de Baets M. Inflammation, depressive symptomtology, and coronary artery disease. Psychosomatic Medicine 2000 Sep-Oct;62(5):601-5.

Appels A. Inflammation and the mental state before an acute coronary event. Annals of Medicine 1999 Apr;31 Suppl 1:41-4.

Other Chronic Diseases

Akash MS, Rehman K, Chen S. Role of inflammatory mechanisms in pathogenesis of type 2 diabetes mellitus. Journal of Cellular Biochemistry 2012 Sep 18. [epub ahead of print]

Johnson AR, Milner JJ, Makowski L. The inflammation highway: metabolism accelerates inflammatory traffic in obesity. Immunological Reviews 2012 Sep;249(1):218-38.

Romeo GR, Lee J, Shoelson SE. Metabolic syndrome, insulin resistance, and roles of inflammation--mechanisms and therapeutic targets. Arteriosclersis, Thrombosis and Vascular Biology 2012 Aug;32(8):1771-6.

Calle MC, Fernandez ML. Inflammation and type 2 diabetes. Diabetes & Metabolism 2012 Jun;38(3):183-91.

Arcidiacono B, Iiritano S, Nocera A, Possidente K, Nevolo MT, Ventura V, Foti D, Chiefari E, Brunetti A. Insulin resistance and cancer risk: an overview of the pathogenetic mechanisms. Experimental Diabetes Research 2012; 2012: 789174 [article number in online journal]

Salim S, Chugh G, Asghar M. Inflammation in anxiety. Advances in Protein Chemistry and Structural Biology 2012; 88:1-25.

Teixeira-Lemos E, Nunes S, Teixeira F, Reis F. Regular physical exercise training assists in preventing type 2 diabetes development: focus on its antioxidant and anti-inflammatory properties. Cardiovascular Diabetology 2011 Jan 28;10:12.

Grammas P. Neurovascular dysfunction, inflammation and endothelial activation: implications for the pathogenesis of Alzheimer's disease. Journal of Neuroinflammation 2011 Mar 25;8:26.

Sastre M, Richardson JC, Gentleman SM, Brooks DJ. Inflammatory risk factors and pathologies associated with Alzheimer's disease. Current Alzheimer Research 2011 Mar;8(2):132-41.

Family Relationships

Books

Gottman, J. M. The Science of Trust: Emotional Attunement for Couples. New York: W. W. Norton & Company, 2011.

Gottman, J.M. & Silver, N. *The Seven Principles for Making Marriage Work*; New York: Crown Publishing, 1999.

Hart, Betty, and Todd R. Risley. *Meaningful Differences in the Everyday Experience of American Children.* Foreword by Lois Bloom. Baltimore, Maryland: Paul H. Brookes Publishing Co, 1995.

Wilson, B.J., & Gottman, J.M., (1995). Marital interaction and parenting. In M.H. Bornstein (Ed.), *Handbook of Parenting,* Vol. 4, Applied and practical parenting, pp. 33-55. (A second edition of this resource has been published in 2012)

Gottman, John M. A Multidemensional Approach to Couples. In F. Kaslow and T. Patterson (Eds.), Comprehensive Handbook of Psychotherapy, Vol. 2, Cognitive-behavioral approaches, 355-372. New York: John Wiley & Sons, 2002.

Journal and Other Articles

Cummings EM, George MR, McCoy KP, Davies PT. Interparental conflict in kindergarten and adolescent adjustment: prospective investigation of emotional security as an explanatory mechanism. Child Development 2012 Sep-Oct;83(5):1703-15.

George MR, Koss KJ, McCoy KP, Cummings EM, Davies PT. Examining the family context and relations with attitudes to school and scholastic competence. Advances in School Mental Health Promotion 2011 Oct;3(4):51-62.

Waters SF, Virmani EA, Thompson RA, Meyer S, Raikes HA, Jochem R. Emotion regulation and attachment: unpacking two constructs and their association. Journal of Psychopathological Behavioral Assessment 2010 Mar;32(1):37-47.

DeBoard-Lucas RL, Fosco GM, Raynor SR, Grych JH. Interparental conflict in context: exploring relations between parenting processes and children's conflict appraisals. Journal of Clinical Child and Adolescent Psychology 2010;39(2):163-75.

Kinsfogel KM, Grych JH. Interparental conflict and adolescent dating relationships: integrating cognitive, emotional, and peer influences. Journal of Family Psychology 2004 Sep;18(3):505-15.

Felitti VJ, Anda RF, Nordenberg D, Williamson DF, Spitz AM, Edwards V, Koss MP, Marks JS. Relationship of childhood abuse and household dysfunction to many of the leading causes of death in adults: The Adverse Childhood Experiences (ACE) Study. American Journal of Preventive Medicine 1998;14:245–258.

Gottman, J.M., Hooven, C., & Katz, L. Parental meta-emotion structure predicts family and child outcomes. Journal of Cognition and Emotion 1995; 9: 229-264.

Katz, L.F., and Gottman, J.M. Patterns of marital interaction and children's emotional development. In R.D. Parke and S.G. Kellam (Eds.), Exploring Family Relationships with Other Social Contexts, Ch. 3, pp. 49-74, Hillsdale, NJ: Lawrence Erlbaum. 1994.

Katz, L.F., and Gottman, J. Marital discord and child outcomes: A social psychophysiological approach. In J. Garber and K. Dodge (Eds.), The development of emotion regulation and dysregulation. Cambridge studies in social and emotional development, p. 129-155. New York: Cambridge University Press, 1991.

Interpersonal Relationships

Books

Daniel Goleman. *The Brain and Emotional Intelligence: New Insights.* Northhampton, MA: More Than Sound, 2011. An e-book.

Williams, Redford, MD, and Virginia Williams PhD. *Lifeskills: 8 Simple Ways to Build Stronger Relationships, Communicate More Clearly, Improve Your Health.* New York: Three Rivers Press, 1998.

Daniel Goleman. *Emotional Intelligence: Why It Can Matter More than IQ.* New York: Bantam, 1995.

Stress

Books

Thomas Steckler, N. H. Kalin. JMHM Reul. *Handbook of Stress and the Brain* (Two Volume Set). Part 1: The Neurobiology of Stress. Part 2: Stress: Integrative and Clinical Aspects. Elsevier Science, 2005.

Sapolsky, Robert M. *Why Zebras Don't Get Ulcers: The Acclaimed Guide to Stress, Stress-Related Disorders and Coping.* Third edition. New York: Henry Holt and Company, 2004.

McEwen, B.S. *The End of Stress as We Know It.* New York: Dana Press, 2002. (Available as an e-book.)

Benson, Herbert, MD, with Miriam Z. Klipper. *The Relaxation Response.* Revised edition. New York: HarperCollins Publishers, Inc., 2000.

Eliot, Dr. Robert S., MD, and Dennis L. Breo. *Is It Worth Dying For? How to Make Stress Work for You—Not Against You.* New York: Bantam Publishing, 1984.

Journal Articles

Rosenkranz MA, Davidson RJ, Maccoon DG, Sheridan JF, Kalin NH, Lutz A. A comparison of mindfulness-based stress reduction and an active control in modulation of neurogenic inflammation. Brain Behavior and Immunity 2012 Oct 22. [Epub ahead of print]

Bevans M, Sternberg EM. Caregiving burden, stress, and health effects among family caregivers of adult cancer patients. JAMA. 2012 Jan 25;307(4):398-403.

Thayer JF, Verkuil B, Brosschot JF, Kampschroer K, West A, Sterling C, Christie IC, Abernethy DR, Sollers JJ, Cizza G, Marques AH, Sternberg EM. Effects of the physical work environment on physiological measures of stress. Eur J Cardiovasc Prev Rehabil. 2010 Aug;17(4):431-9.

Silverman MN, Heim CM, Nater UM, Marques AH, Sternberg EM. Neuroendocrine and immune contributors to fatigue. PM & R: The Journal of Injury, Function and Rehabilitation 2010 May;2(5):338-46.

Chandola T, Britton A, Brunner E, Hemingway H, Malik M, Kumari M, Badrick E, Kivimaki M, Marmot M. Work stress and coronary heart disease: what are the mechanisms? European Heart Journal 2008 Mar;29(5):640-8.

Tait AS, Butts CL, Sternberg EM. The role of glucocorticoids and progestins in inflammatory, autoimmune, and infectious disease. Journal of Leukocyte Biology 2008 Oct;84(4):924-31.

McEwen, B.S. and Wingfield, J.C. The concept of allostasis in biology and biomedicine. *Hormones & Behavior 2003;* 43:2-15.

Website

Relaxation Techniques for Health: An Introduction.
http://nccam.nih.gov/health/stress/relaxation.htm
        Information and resources from the National Center for Complementary and Alternative Medicine, National Institutes of Health.

ONLINE VIDEOS

There are many online videos that outline effective techniques for such things as relaxation, stress reduction, cardiovascular exercise and anger management.

Acknowledgements

I'm very thankful for the opportunity to have served the many patients who have shared their stories with me, both individually and within the group format. The power of the group setting is in the microcosm of life created in the presence of others. This allows members to work on problems simultaneously, at whatever level of insight, openness, maturity, and growth they are experiencing at that time. This book has grown with the groups over the years and is a product of specific requests from the original members. The individual stories are of real people; of course, the names have been changed except where noted.

Thanks and gratitude extend to Mary Abbott Waite, an experienced medical writer, who assisted not only as editor, but in building the structure and foundation for the book, then prepared it for publication. She did this in spite of the many other significant jobs her loyal customers have given her.

Thanks to my wife, Flo, and my family for their patience during the time taken to complete this project over these many years. Flo has been an essential partner and adviser whose opinions, critiques, and encouragement have influence throughout the book.

About the Author

Jack Dawson, MD is the Director of Cardiac Rehabilitation at the Fuqua Heart Center of Piedmont Hospital in Atlanta, Georgia. He has been a practicing clinician in Cardiology for forty years in Atlanta and has pioneered in the use of social and psychological support in conjunction with physical rehabilitation in the secondary and primary prevention of chronic disease. He currently practices with Piedmont Heart Institute at Piedmont Hospital. He is a graduate of the Medical College of Georgia and completed his Cardiology Fellowship at Emory University School of Medicine Hospitals in Atlanta.

www.ingramcontent.com/pod-product-compliance
Lightning Source LLC
Chambersburg PA
CBHW062049270326
41931CB00013B/3005